THE
FERMENTATION
KITCHEN

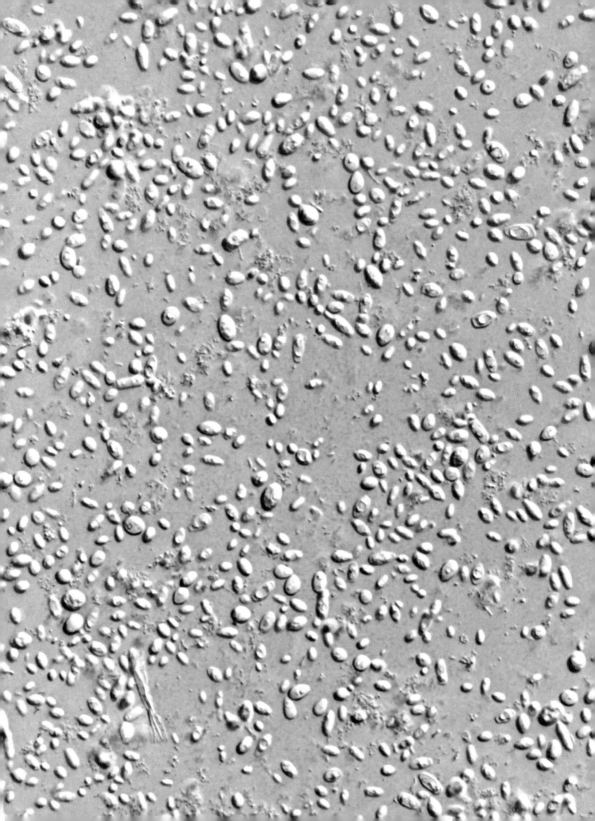

SAM COOPER

THE
FERMENTATION
KITCHEN

Recipes and techniques for kimchi, kombucha, kōji, and more

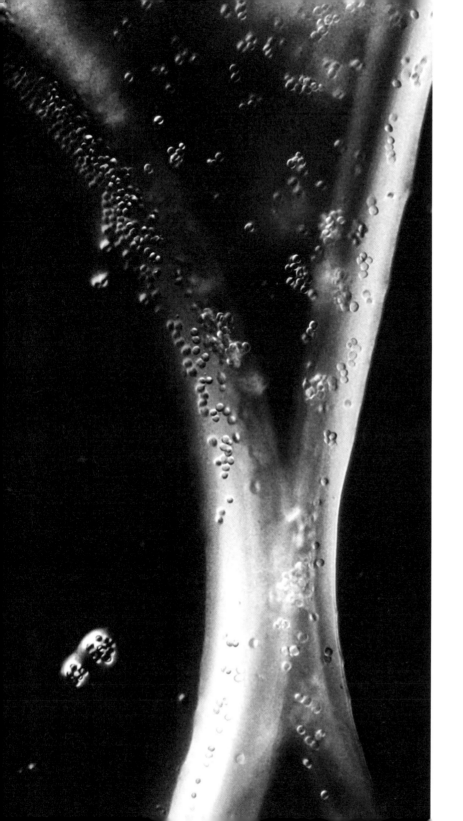

CONTENTS

Previous A micro shot of yeast and bacteria cells in kombucha. **Left** A micro shot of yeast cells.

I've always been obsessed with food. As a child, my first true love was cheese—the more brutally funky, the better. It's no surprise that I fell into cheffing, but it took many years before I came to realize that fermentation lay behind every great flavor I loved: the wine in stock, tangy cheeses, yogurts and crème fraîche, cultured butters, pickled vegetables, fruity vinegars, sauerkraut, and kimchi. Increasingly, I noticed chefs from cuisines across the world using tamari or soy sauce in their stock, mirin in their sauces, and miso in everything from mashed potatoes to sticky toffee pudding.

Many years later, having tested techniques from all over the world and learned from some of the best fermenters alive today, it is my honor to share with you a book full of flavor you won't find anywhere else—customized and adapted for every kitchen of every shape and size.

You might notice that throughout this book, I photograph making ferments everywhere. From a small rented kitchen to a new white one, and from windowsills to desks and offices—the list goes on. I wrote this book in the middle of moving house and building a kitchen. If that doesn't give you the confidence that you, too, can make every recipe no matter the kind of kitchen you have, I don't know what will.

In this book, I will outline the fermentation processes for a handful of my favorite microbes, along with recipes that I hope will inspire you to use these ferments in everyday cooking. I've grouped these recipes into three broad categories, based on the dominant microbes responsible for them: bacteria, yeast, and mold. These categories take you from the simplest life form to the most complex.

While most of these recipes may seem remarkably simple, my hope is that you will progress through them, picking up a solid understanding of each type of fermentation. The book is structured to take you through ferments from the quickest to those that will take more time. Once you've gained this basic intuition, it will form a bedrock for the more complex methods, such as

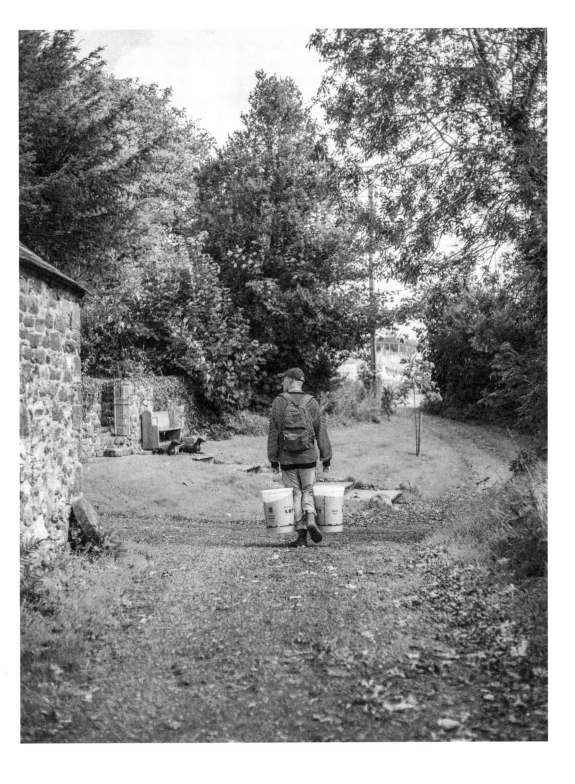

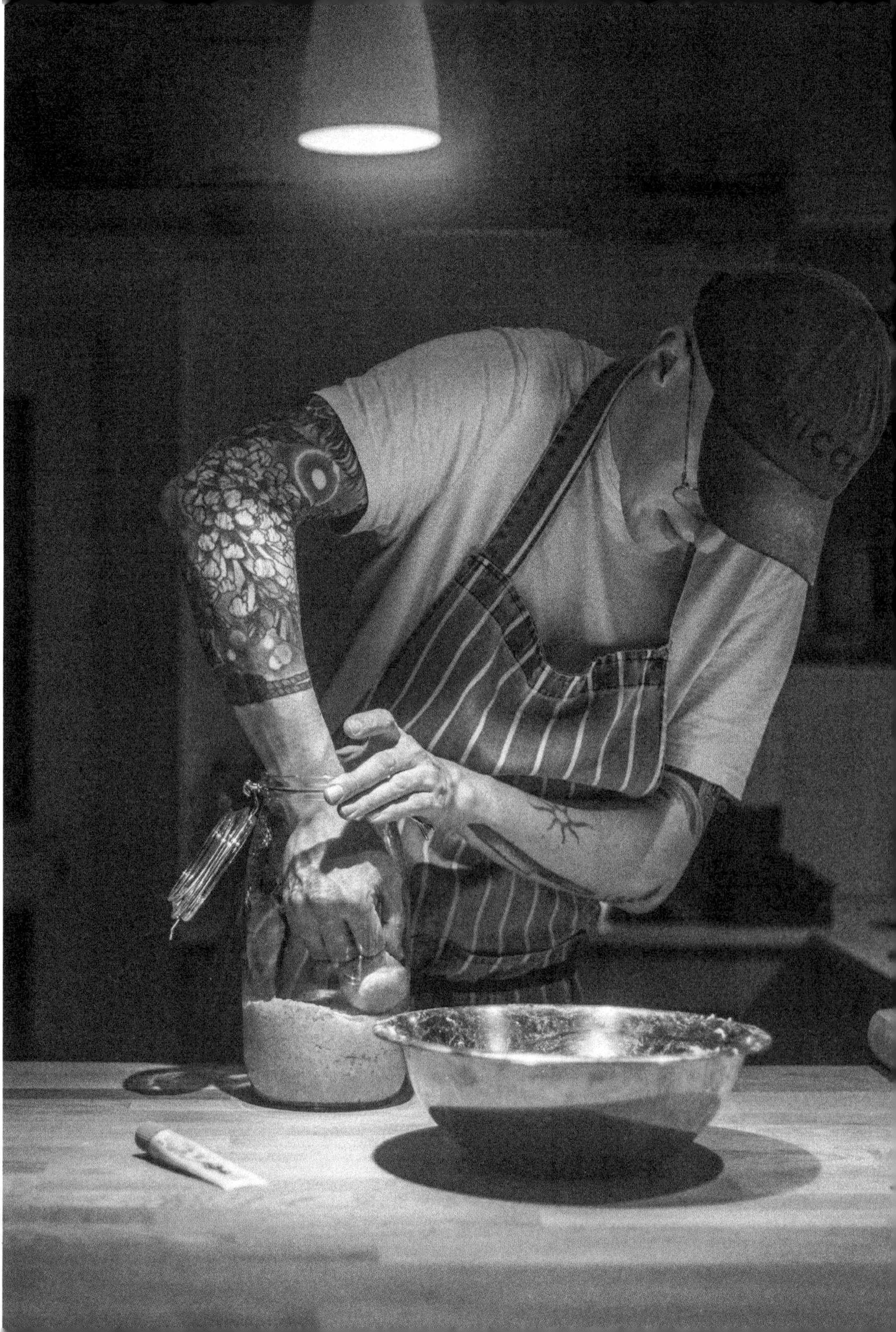

homemade miso (see pp.191–197) and shoyu (see pp.202–207). The focus of these techniques will be vegetables, fruit, grains, legumes, and fungi, with a handful of dairy recipes. This is because I am a gardener, and these often-overlooked ingredients naturally find themselves at the foundation of my work. Plants are also less bioavailable and digestible than other foods, having evolved ingenious defense mechanisms in place of being able to run away. Through fermentation, I will show you a natural microbial solution to breaking through these defenses to make some of the most delicious, diverse, and healthy foods you can.

I will help you understand the nature of microorganisms by providing context, technique, and in-depth instructions. Each recipe serves as a template, with follow-up examples that demonstrate the breadth and possibilities of your own creative endeavors. By the time you've finished reading this book, you'll have the knowledge to set out on your own microbial adventure and discover flavors you cannot find anywhere else and the confidence to create your own recipes to share with your family and friends.

The section on cooking with fermented foods (see pp.56–61) brings together useful guidance on how to use ferments in everyday meals. By putting taste, texture, and aroma at the forefront of your cooking, you can create food that cannot be bought from supermarkets or replicated in factories. This is food marked by hands— and, in some cases, by the very microbes living on your hands, too.

So, without further ado, please join me as I guide you through a world of time and taste.

Microbes are everywhere. They are all over and within you. They sustain you—and the world we live in. These tiny and diverse species remain largely a mystery, but the more we learn about them, the more we realize that nothing makes sense without them.

A MICROBIAL WORLD

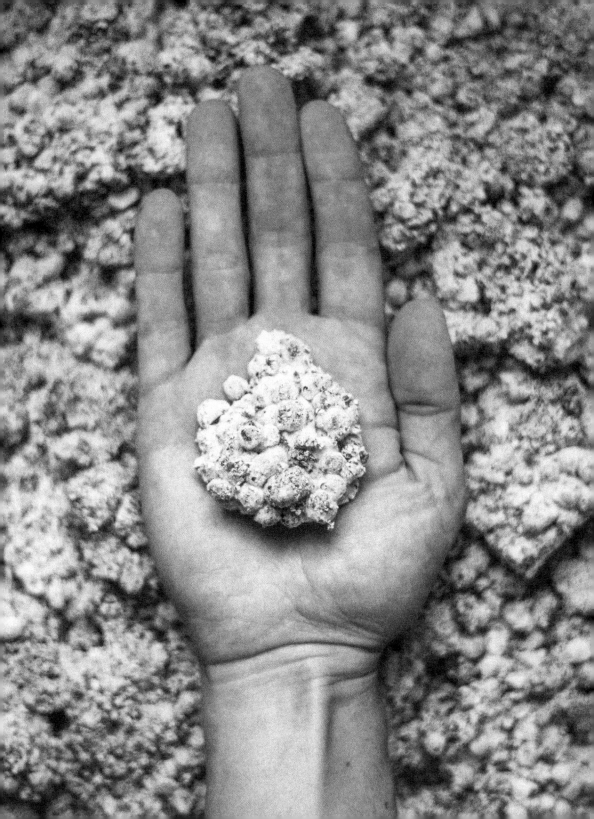

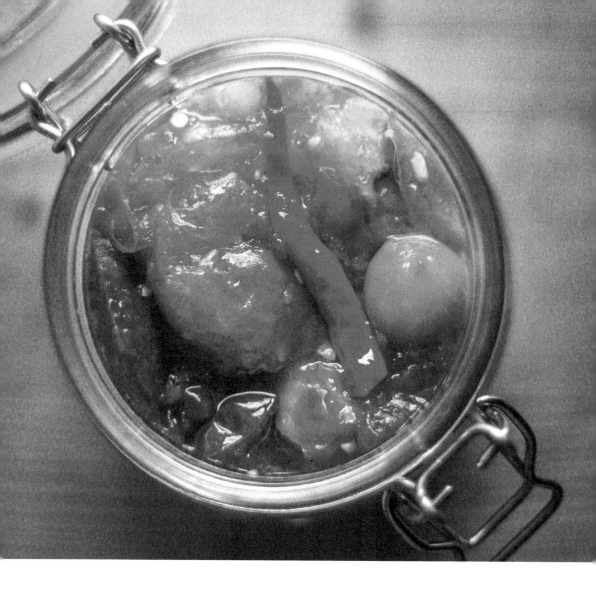

ENTER THE
MICROCOSMOS

A medley of fermenting
tomatoes and chilies,
where infusion, microbes,
enzymes, and acids
unlock unique flavors.

The only time in my life when I wasn't working in kitchens,
I spent five years in academia, practicing fine art. While there
were many aspects of the institution I clashed with, among
its long-lasting gifts was an idea that has stuck with me:
lenses of observation. In art, there is specific emphasis on
using our sense of sight, and sometimes hearing and touch,
in order to observe and interact with the world around us
with active intention. For me, having lived and breathed food
all my life (in both the kitchen and the garden), taste, smell,
and touch became my lenses of choice. Through the act of
eating, we are able to detect the chemical and nutritional
make-up of an ingredient: we can experience sunlight in the
form of ripened sugars; aromatic compounds that indicate
bioavailability of nutrients and minerals; and texture—both
with our hands and in the act of chewing—that can cause
pleasure or repulsion.

Our senses give us a glimpse into a world far too small
for us to see and too quiet to hear: a world belonging to
microbes. By the time we eat it, a single nutrient has been
on a journey from solid rock. It was released into soil by
fungi and algae, often working together in symbiosis, and
from there it was made available for plants by the microbes
living in the rhizosphere, a living trade network around
plants' roots. Leaves, stem, flower, and fruit, all flushed with
nutrients, are then harvested and prepared by us. In doing
so, we experience this microscopic adventure through
taste and aroma. In fact, our senses are so acute, our
olfactory system alone can detect the bonds between
molecules for every known substance we've ever tasted.
There are, however, techniques we can use in the
preparation of our ingredients that introduce additional
microbes to unlock even more flavor, increase
bioavailability of nutrients, and even neutralize toxins.

INTRODUCING FERMENTATION

Fermentation is the process of subjecting ingredients to
certain conditions that are favorable to the microorganisms
that benefit us. Often, this involves the sealing away of food
inside vessels while time passes, allowing metamorphosis to
take place. Much like opening a perfectly ripe piece of fruit
and peering inside, there is a degree of magic in

fermentation that pulls us into the here and now. While we may be in charge of the conditions to which we subject our ingredients, the transformations they provoke dispel our expectations. Unlike cooking, where the process leads you to know, more or less, what to expect when you take that first bite, the reality of opening a jar of fermented ingredients can be very far from our expectations.

Fermentation requires a shift in thinking. In cooking, we're used to straightforward, chemistrylike math. X heat for Y time = deliciousness. Fermentation is a biological process—one which can offer incredible results—and the math is more akin to quantum computing. A set of ingredients, given the right conditions, can yield more than the sum of its parts. Sometimes, $1 + 1 = 3$.

HUMAN VESSEL

Most things with an inside and outside can form a vessel for fermentation, including you.

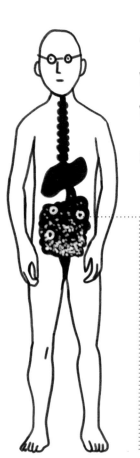

THE WONDER*FUL* WORK OF *MICROBES*

These tireless, unseen creatures are everywhere, within and all over every part of us. If you think of a human as a fleshy tube (which I often do), lined on the outside by skin and the inside by our digestive tract, then you'll find microbes teeming on every tiny bit of us. From a microbial perspective, we fleshy tubes are like TARDISes, far bigger on the inside than out. Our gut alone, if unfolded, would cover a space of 344 square feet (32 square meters), housing more bacteria than there are stars in our galaxy. With this ample room providing miniature ecosystems all over us, it's no wonder that we actually house more microbes than our own cells. We're in constant exchange with these microbes, as

Your gut microbiome is a form of fermentation you carry with you, unlocking nutrients your body cannot unlock alone.

they are with one another, providing us with access to nutrients that we couldn't digest without them. And, from one fleshy tube to another, we don't just live in a microbe's world, we are an indistinguishable part of it. Luckily, they're far more helpful than we often give them credit for.

What makes microbes so useful is their ability to unlock nutrients by producing enzymes (more on those later), as well as the effects of their ecosystem on foods. Throughout this book, you will be dipping into two types of fermentation: primary and secondary.

PRIMARY FERMENTATION

This is when microbes actively live within a substance and break it down with enzymes.

CHANGES IN MOLECULAR STRUCTURE

Given ideal conditions and time, microbes alter the molecular structure of the food.

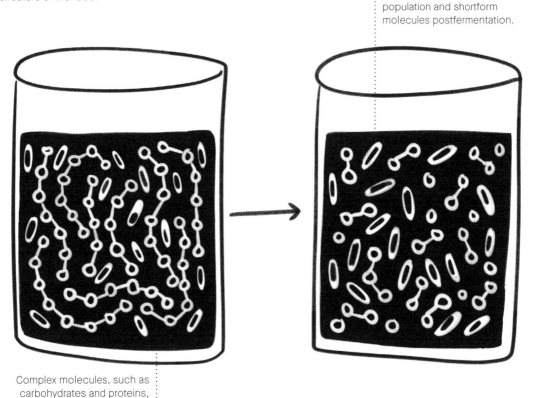

An increased microbial population and shortform molecules postfermentation.

Complex molecules, such as carbohydrates and proteins, prior to fermentation.

FERMENTATION AND HEALTH

There are a lot of health claims that float around the subject of fermentation. While I have no doubt fermentation is healthy for you—we humans have been doing it long enough to figure that out—I'm skeptical of the beneficial impact of any single dietary alteration. Sticking to a wide variety of ingredients, eating seasonally, avoiding junk food and excess—all have an accumulating effect on our health, and fermented foods play their part. Through fermentation, we can unlock nutrients and produce enzymes that our bodies alone cannot. This means fermented ingredients often have more bioavailability compared to their unfermented counterparts. There are also bacteria that can survive passage through our stomachs and adhere to our intestines, where they form a symbiotic part of our microbiome. But I won't sell you the message that fermented foods have an especially significant role in human health any more so than including lots of dietary fibre and staying clear of pesticides and antibiotics.. I'm a chef after all, not a doctor. So my aim is to share with you some of the fermentation techniques I use to unlock incredible flavor. By all means, eat fermented food, but do so as part of a balanced and delicious diet. That's what I do, anyway.

SECONDARY FERMENTATION

There are three types of secondary fermentation. One is when we use one set of microbes to produce the conditions for another set of microbes—for example, using yeast to ferment sugars into ethanol, then turning the ethanol into acetic acid (vinegar) with bacteria.

The second type is when we load an ingredient with enzymes from one set of microbes, then mix those with another ingredient. While there's often nothing technically alive left from the first round of fermentation, the following microbes can take advantage of the first's enzymes and unlock flavor in a whole new ingredient (one that might not house favorable conditions for the microbes themselves)—for example, in miso (see pp.191–197).

Finally, we can even combine these approaches by mixing the enzymes of one ferment with another ferment, or in the case of wine, age a ferment long after microbial activity has died off, allowing the leftover enzymes to continue floating around, unlocking flavor. You'll see this process in action in a few of the recipes later in the book.

While it isn't hugely important to distinguish between these approaches, it's nice to know.

My aim is to share with you some of the fermentation techniques I use to unlock incredible flavor.

TWO STAGES OF FERMENTATION

Fermentation is often a step in preparing an ingredient for further microbial alteration.

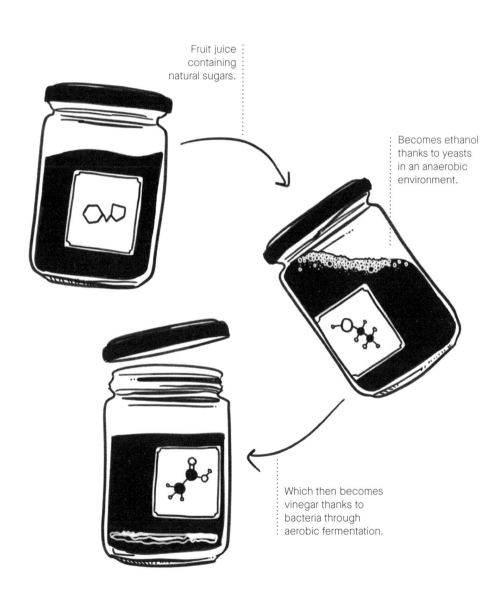

Fruit juice containing natural sugars.

Becomes ethanol thanks to yeasts in an anaerobic environment.

Which then becomes vinegar thanks to bacteria through aerobic fermentation.

JADAM

My first interaction with microbes was the rigorous cleaning and sanitization of the kitchens in restaurants I worked at. Like a lot of people, I assumed all microorganisms were bad and out to get us. When people find out I ferment, the first thing they ask is, "Aren't you scared you'll poison yourself?" These days, I'm far friendlier with microbes. The subtle shift in my perspective started when I first met Nigel Palmer, a gardener from the US who introduced me to the South Korean farming practice called JADAM. You can think of JADAM as many things, but essentially it is fermentation for garden

plants. The idea is harnessing the power of microbes to make natural amendments and foliar sprays from weeds and foraged ingredients in an attempt to have a garden or farm "gut biome" that mimics the ecosystems found in similar natural settings, such as woodlands or meadows. But more importantly, some of these concoctions are alive with microbes. I distinctly remember Nigel showed me a beautiful, healthy pear tree on his land. The year before, it was dying of a fungal disease that had run rampant. Instead of attacking the disease with a fungicide, Nigel treated it with a microbially rich, homemade foliar spray. This influx of

friendly microbes acted as a source of competition for the fungus, knocking it back into place. The important part is, when kept in check by the competition of a healthy microbiome, the very same fungus that was killing the tree is part of a beneficial and supportive symbiosis. The point in this story is to highlight that the most important thing to cultivate when starting out with this book is mindset. If we learn to live with microbes, we can thrive from the benefits.

ENZYMES

Enzymes are proteins that break down substances and build others. We all know how powerful this is; after all, our very DNA is formed from chains of proteins. Our bodies produce some enzymes in order to digest the food we eat, but microbes are the true masters. As previously mentioned, our gut microbiome is a community of microorganisms located in our intestinal tract, which forms our very own bioreactor, providing us with access to a whole host of nutrients. By producing enzymes, these microbes make nutrients bioavailable to us that would otherwise go to waste.

Through fermentation, we can harness the power of enzymes to make food more nutritionally available to us before even eating it. But the uses don't stop there. About 60 percent of enzymes used in industry are produced by fungi, as well as all citric acid in carbonated drinks. The "bio" element of biological detergent is synthesized from an enzyme produced by Aspergillus, a genus of fungi. And in 2017, researchers from China and Pakistan reported they had discovered a fungus, *Aspergillus tubingensis*, that was even breaking down plastic at a landfill site in Islamabad, Pakistan (Ekanayaka A. H., Tibpromma S., Dai D., Xu R., Suwannarach N., Stephenson S. L., Dao C., Karunarathna S. C., "A Review of the Fungi that Degrade Plastic"). While not as tasty, this last example truly shows the power of enzymes. With them, microbes hold every key to unlocking the world at a fundamental level. And through fermentation, we can direct the actions of microbes to suit our specific needs.

PROTEINS AND ENZYMES

Enzymes are biocatalysts that speed up biochemical reactions.

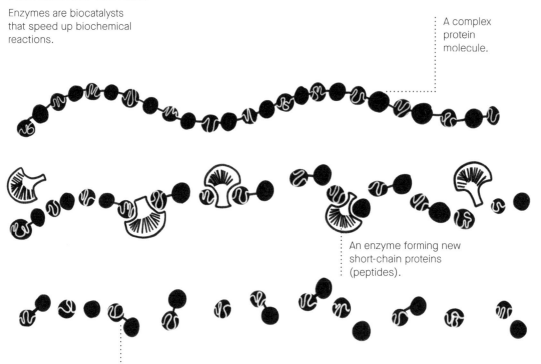

A complex protein molecule.

An enzyme forming new short-chain proteins (peptides).

A short-chain protein (peptide), which we can taste as a range of flavors.

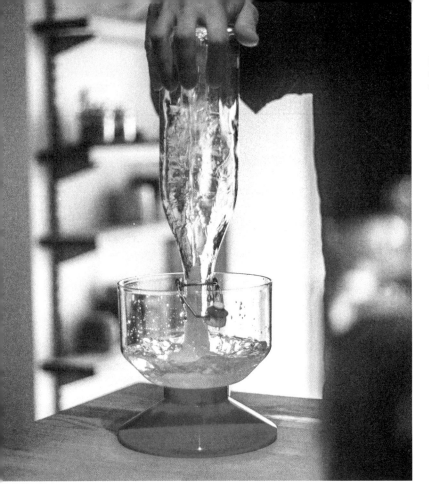

Cultures around the world fall into two categories: those
with a phobia of microbes, and those which have embraced
them for thousands of years.

I come from a culture where most people think bacteria
means death, but they push such thoughts into the far
recesses of their minds as they gleefully spoon yogurt onto
their breakfast, nibble on some cheese late at night, or take

SAFETY

that first intoxicating sip of alcohol. For many, they argue that these foods are trustworthy because they're made by professionals wearing lab coats and hairnets in industrial kitchens and factories. They probably even have clipboards. These people harness the power of lab-produced microbes and sterilized ingredients, but the reality is that we humans have been fermenting for thousands of years, long before hairnets and clipboards.

CLEAN*ING* VS. *SANITIZATION*

Fermentation is a living process, and one that can sometimes go wrong. This might be as simple as a ferment stalling, or suffering from a false start, or it could be worse. Always take care when selecting, cleaning, and preparing your ingredients, as well as cleaning and sanitizing your equipment. The difference here is that cleaning involves the removal of dirt or debris; sanitizing is the process of removing most microbiology from your equipment. There is a range of sanitizing products available in home-brew supply stores and online that will help you make sure your work surface, utensils, and equipment are all ready for use. (Always follow the product instructions.)

Caution, in due amount, is important when approaching fermentation, but do not worry. In the following pages, I will outline the factors and considerations that act as our tools of control in the process of fermentation. Most importantly, and I will say this multiple times throughout this book, weigh ingredients properly and never be tempted to lower the amount of salt in a recipe. That, paired with good cleaning and sanitization, should be enough to reassure you that it is possible to keep the following dangerous bacteria at bay.

SANITIZING AT HOME

A simple hot wash in the dishwasher can be used to sanitize, if you have one. Failing that, you can place glass, metal, and ceramic equipment in the oven and dry-sterilize them at 325°F (160°C) for 2 hours. For materials that will burn or melt—such as fabric, wood, or plastic—put them in boiling water or steam them for 2 minutes. (This can also be done with metal and ceramic equipment, but take extra care with glass, as it can shatter.)

CLOSTRIDIUM BOTULINUM

A rod-shaped, anaerobic bacteria most commonly found in soil and sediment. It produces botulism, a rare but dangerous toxin that causes reversible flaccid paralysis.

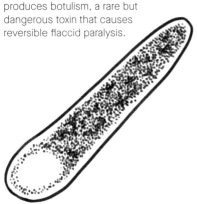

CLOSTRIDIUM BOTULINUM

The big bad one that most people worry about is *Clostridium botulinum*, the bacteria responsible for botulism. This rare and potent toxin is known for its uses in the world of beauty as botox and is most commonly found in soil. Botulism didn't capture the fears of people around the world until the advent of canning. This process involves sealing food in an airtight container and heating it up to sterilize the contents within. However, if canning is done incorrectly, the bacteria can survive and thrive in the absence of oxygen. The danger here is the lack of acidity. Botulinum cannot tolerate conditions that have a pH of 4.5 or lower, a sustained temperature of 140°F (60°C) or above, and has difficulty in fluids with a salt concentration of 5 percent or higher. In ferments like lacto fermentation (see p.66), acidity increases as the ferment ages. Starting with a 2 percent salinity is enough to hinder *Clostridium botulinum* while the ferment naturally sours. On day 3, I check to make sure the pH is below 5. By full maturity, it is considered safe below 4.6.

SALMONELLA

Another rod-shaped bacteria that's responsible for thousands of cases of food poisoning each year.

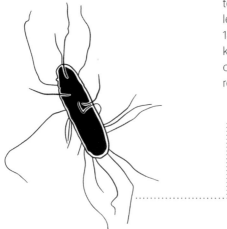

SALMONELLA

Most often associated with raw milk and poultry, the salmonella bacteria can also survive on unwashed fruit and vegetables. The first line of defense is to sanitize the station between the handling of such food groups to prevent cross-contamination. When fermenting, salt levels of 10 percent, or several minutes at temperatures of 140–149°F (60–65°C), such as during yogurt-making, will kill off salmonella. Never use the same utensil for unfinished or raw ingredients and a finished ferment, as this can reintroduce the bacteria.

Salmonella has several peritrichous flagella— long, hairlike filaments it uses to move.

MOLDS AND OTHERS

In fermentation, we often produce ideal environments for the many thousands of varieties of molds and pathogenic bacteria (such as *E. coli*) to thrive. In cases like these, sanitization is our first priority, especially if you handle raw meat and animal products in the same space. The most effective counter to *E. coli* is the thorough cleaning of vegetables and fruit in cold water prior to fermentation. For mold, a combination of salt and disturbance is enough to interrupt growth. Mold will appear on the surface of ferments, so stirring or even shaking a ferment once a day will stop mold from gaining a foothold.

ESCHERICHIA COLI

There are numerous *E. coli* (*Escherichia coli*) bacteria living in your gut microbiome that cause no harm, but some strains can make you sick.

Small, hairlike structures on the outside are called pili and help the bacteria attach to surfaces.

Coli have multiple flagella distributed over the cell surface that rotate and allows the bacterium to swim.

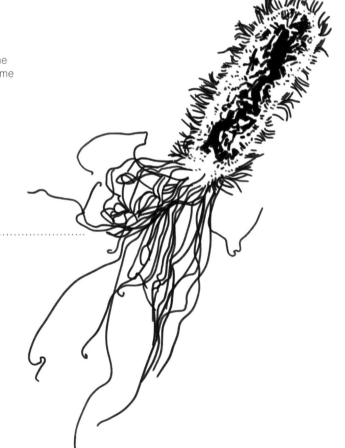

A MICROBIAL WORLD

Carbon dioxide bubbles rushing upward through fermenting tomato juices as bacteria and yeast feed on natural sugars.

LIVING FOODS

There is an often-overlooked advantage that fermented foods have over other foods, such as canned and pickled: they're alive. In canned food, the attempt to pasteurize the content leaves no competition for pathogens, which are then free to take over if the correct timings and temperature were not achieved. Fermented foods thrive with their diverse, healthy populations of microbes, which simply overpower intruders.

We also use techniques to push the odds in our favor. Adding salt at the beginning of the process hinders unpleasant microbes while benefiting others. Controlling oxygen, temperature, moisture, and acidity are all handy tricks to improve our chances of a successful ferment. Finally, once we know a ferment has gone well, we often use a percentage of that mature microbial population to inoculate a new batch in a method called "backslopping." (Sexy, right?) This technique floods the new ferment with friendly, healthy microbes right from the get-go, leaving no chance for anything else to slip in early and take over.

Above all else, trust your nose. As I mentioned before, your sense of smell is your window into the world of microorganisms. Most ferments have their own interesting, powerful aromas, but if it smells bad, then you should always throw it out and start again. Never take the risk. If you aren't sure, consult the troubleshooting section in this book (see pp.214–217).

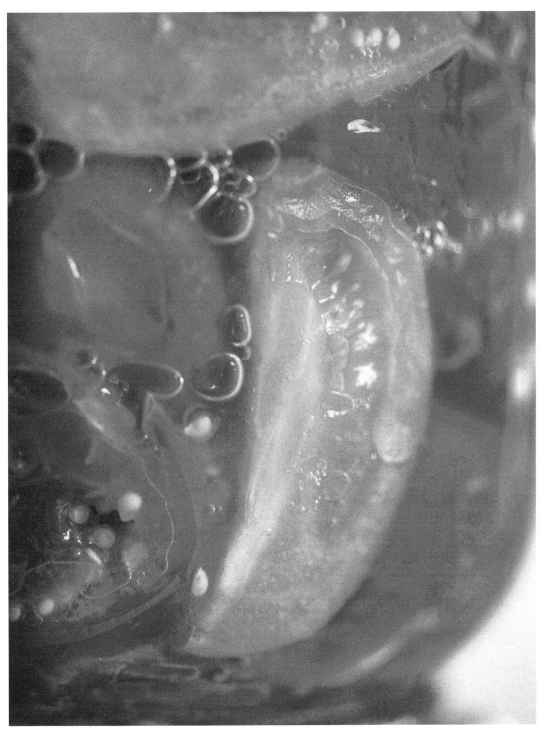

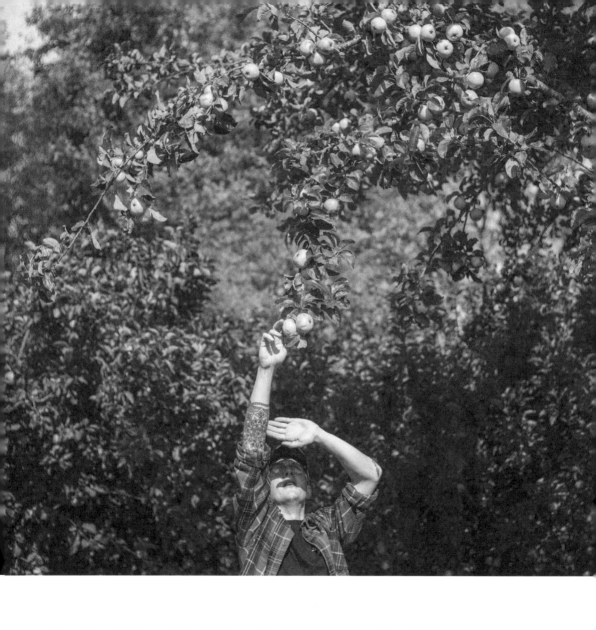

NAVIGATING
FERMENTATION

In working with microbes, we can only set the stage and wait. It is a slow, nurturing process, more similar to farming or shepherding a flock than cooking.

It is important to think of microbes as a living community that acts as a whole and changes over time. You will read a lot about fermentation with high-tech setups and perfectly controlled environments, which are great if you're trying to replicate a particular flavor or certain commercial standard. I, however, revel in the seasonality and vintage of fermentation. Much as we celebrate a great year of wine or the appearance of winter cheeses, my approach to fermentation is to work with the seasons and promote naturally ideal conditions. This makes the process far more accessible in the average kitchen and encourages you to adapt to the produce of your region, as well as the conditions you live in.

INGREDIENTS

While it might be possible to ferment anything, not all ingredients are created equal. Some will burst into action, thriving with microbial life, while others will sit there doing nothing. There are a few key things to bear in mind when selecting ingredients, as well as a couple of tricks to help you with those that are less than perfect.

SEASONAL

Pick the ingredients that are in season. Not only will these be fresh, ripe, and brimming with microbes, they are also most likely grown in the most natural setup. When farmers use techniques to speed up the ripening process, or even produce or store some ingredients all year round, they might have artificially cheated the clock at a superficial level, but the absence of microbes won't lie.

Not all ingredients are created equal.

ORGANIC

Organic can mean different things in different countries. A general rule in my country (the UK) is that organic farms don't use a lot of the pesticides, fungicides, and chemical fertilizers that are known to inhibit microbial life, but you may need to check what the certification looks like for you. There's a reason organic food often looks knobby and has a shorter shelf life: the same microbes that cause it to spoil are the ones waiting for you to ferment them. The same is true for heirloom varieties. Plants evolved to thrive in a microbe's world, but in recent years we've interrupted that.

CLEAN

While it should be obvious that the ingredients you select should be clean before fermenting, it is just as important that the water is clean. Where I live, tap water is incredibly clean, so I can often get away with using it. But sometimes, tap water is full of many things as part of its sanitation process, and this makes it highly unsuitable to use in fermenting. If this is the case, you can use filtered water as a cost-effective solution, but you may even want to use spring water.

FERMENTATION HEROES

If you've tried a recipe in this book and it struggled to spring into life, there are two small, unassuming ingredients that have never failed to ignite a ferment with microbes: garlic and ginger root. Select whichever one is most suitable as a pairing with the ingredients you wish to ferment (as they will certainly infuse their flavors) and put in a peeled clove of garlic or knob of ginger. Both are loaded with microbes and will act as an inoculant. However, the same rules apply: you will need fresh, organic garlic and ginger for this truly to work.

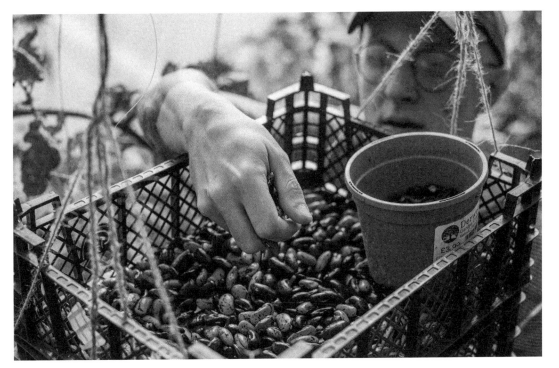

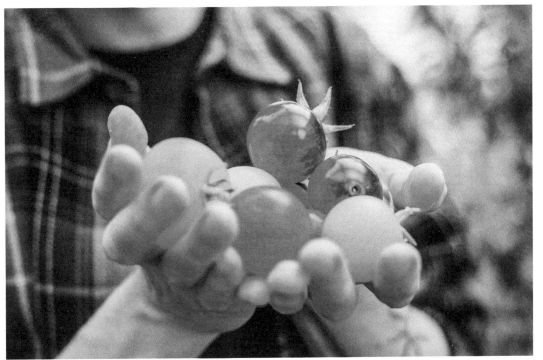

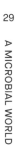

SIZE AND SPEED OF GROWTH

This shows the relative scale of common fermentation microbes. The average growth rate for the bacteria, yeast, and mold featured in this book is 20 minutes, 2 hours, and 2 days respectively.

Lactic acid bacteria 1–1.5µm.

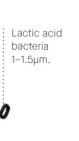

Yeast cell 3–8µm.

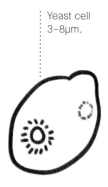

TIME AND TEMPERAT*URE*

In the ancient British orchards, cider is traditionally made in fall. In Japan, sake, which is made from rice harvested in fall, is fermented in the dead of winter. Both processes take advantage of the cold months to slow fermentation down, holding the drinks at each stage of their journey for as long as possible to tease out complex and nuanced flavors. Winter also acts as a reset in nature, killing off or making dormant a lot of pests and diseases that could otherwise cause problems for such a slow and delicate ferment.

At the other end of the spectrum, *Aspergillus oryzae* (see p.161) is a tropical fungus that gives us incredible foods, like miso and soy sauce, and is most suited to the climate of a jungle (or, as it turns out, cooler climates and a hot-water bottle). If we dig a little deeper, we realize that there are many temperatures to consider. For *A. oryzae*, there are different ideal temperatures depending on whether it's being used for a protein-rich ingredient or starch-rich ingredient and another set of temperatures that

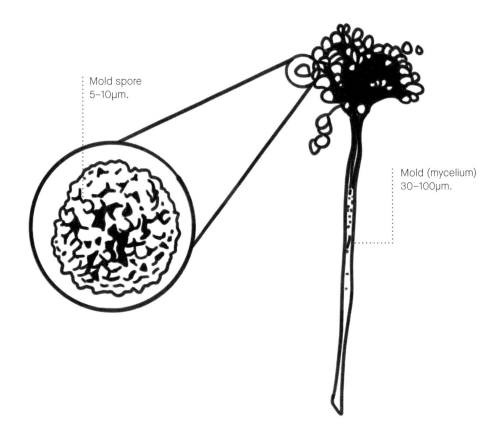

Mold spore
5–10µm.

Mold (mycelium)
30–100µm.

OVEN TEMPERATURES

All temperatures listed in this book in relation to an oven are for a fan/convection oven and should be adjusted accordingly for your oven if using a conventional oven. Note: when using an oven to sterilize equipment, if you use a conventional oven, only use the top shelf to ensure the correct temperature range is achieved.

are better suited to the enzymes it produces. There are even further complications for ferments that work with a host of different microbes all at once.

The following recipes are ordered by the size and speed of the microbes they use, which generally reflects the simplicity of the ferment. Lactic acid bacteria (LAB, see p.64), my bacteria of choice, can quickly overrun its competition, making it very easy to work with. *A. oryzae* (see p.161), a slow-acting fungus, is a more complex life form and takes time. Therefore, there is more we must do to make sure LAB and other quicker organisms don't take over.

For each recipe in this book, I will include both time and temperature, along with tips for how to adjust the recipe if your conditions are different. You can also read more in the section on your fermentation station (see p.54) for how I'd optimize conditions with home setups.

Shaking fermenting
cranberries to agitate
the surface and prevent
mold growth.

FINISHING TEMPERATURE

When activity has come to an end, or a ferment has reached the desired flavor and you want to halt the process, you have a few choices. Most ferments will last in the fridge, in an airtight container, for weeks to months, but some will require freezing, drying, or pasteurization. These all halt microbial activity but in different ways. Freezing will put microbes into a dormant state but preserve the nutrients and enzymes released during fermentation. However, you may quickly run out of room in your freezer, so if you need to store ferments at room temperature, then your other options are to pasteurize or dry them. A lot of fermenters don't like the pasteurization process, as it can denature enzymes, alter flavor, and soften any preserved crunchy ingredients into a mush. Drying can be done seasonally, using the sun and wind, or in a fan oven or dehydrator. Removing the moisture at a low temperature is a great way to slow microbes right down, but you will alter the texture significantly. For some ferments, this is favorable, as it adds crunch or chewiness, but for others, it's a compromise for long-term ambient storage. None are quite as perfect as working with freshly fermented food, but for long-term storage, they serve a purpose.

MOTION

Another tool at our disposal is motion. By mixing a ferment, we can increase the amount of oxygen in a liquid, send surface-dwelling spores to a salty grave, break down ingredients, redistribute enzymes, or disturb the growth of harmful microbes that rely on oxygen before they've even had a chance to appear. For the same reason a pond will turn stagnant but a river stays clear, motion is an important factor in fermentation. If a recipe calls for you to stir something once per week, it's usually for a good reason.

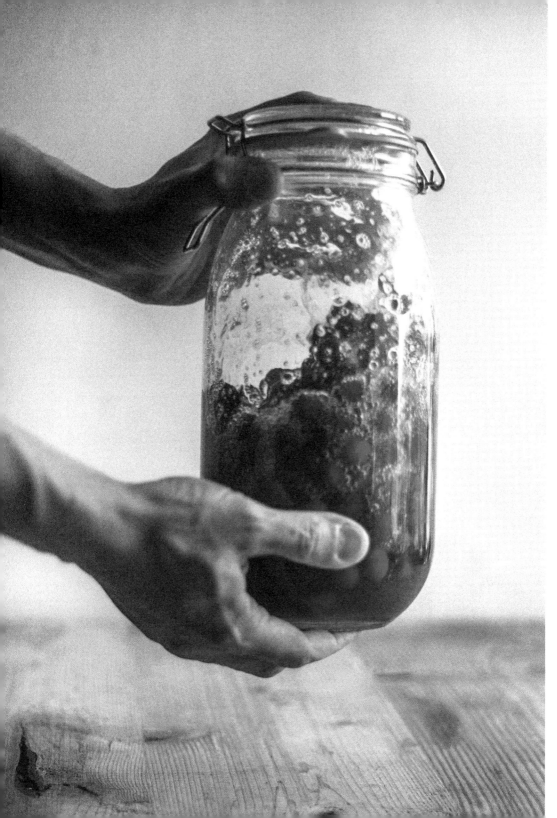

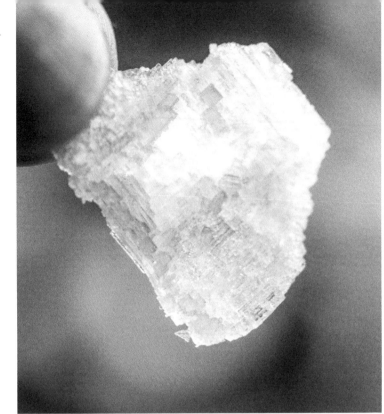

Left A macro of salt crystal structure.

Below Lemons are one of the most acidic naturally occurring foods, making them valuable for fermentation.

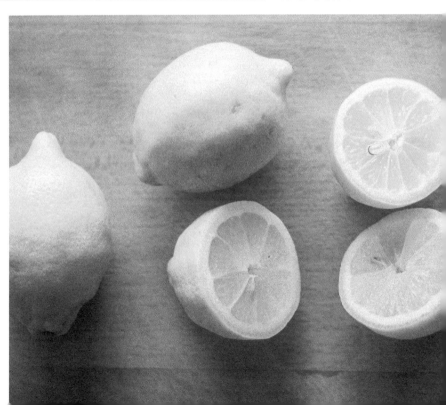

SALT
AND *ACID*

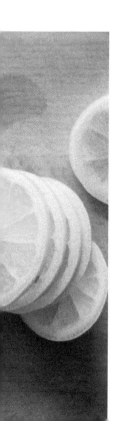

The two major defenses against unwanted—sometimes dangerous—microbes are salt and acid. By harnessing them, we can help protect our ferments from the intrusion of pathogens that could impart unpleasant flavors or make us sick. Salt is often the first line of defense, creating a hostile environment for a lot of harmful microorganisms. This could range from 2 percent for an acidic ferment to 10 percent for something not acidic. The amount of salt is crucial to making sure a ferment is safe to eat, so if you wish to avoid too much salt in your diet, don't be tempted to cut back on the recipe. Instead, reduce how much of the ferment you eat in a sitting. Personally, I'm not a fan of overly salty food, so it is worth remembering that not all salt is created equal. I tend toward milder-tasting salts like Flor de Sal, or a local Welsh salt, Halen Môn. Fine sea salts are commonly used, but make sure they don't include any anticaking agents. I'm sometimes especially naughty and splash out on some smoked salt, which infuses my ferments with additional aroma and depth. The two types of salt to avoid are table salt and iodized salt. Table salt isn't pure salt, and the anticaking agents can mess with your ferments. Iodized salt is fortified with potassium iodide for thyroid health but significantly inhibits microbial activity.

WHAT DOES SALT DO?
The mechanism at play here is exactly the same as salting meat or vegetables ahead of cooking them. The salt draws moisture from the cells, dissolving into it and breaking into ions, which proceed to move inward. Vegetables wrinkle and meat becomes noticeably looser and more jellylike. The same happens to living cells, such as you and I, or microbes. The salt ions draw moisture from the cells until they die, but some microbes have a greater tolerance of this than others. This is why it's important to be exact when measuring salt in fermentation: too much and you'll inhibit activity and flavor; too little and you run the risk of pathogens surviving.

It is important
to know the pH
of your ferments.

WHAT DOES ACID DO?

Acidity is one of the major preserving factors and well-known flavors in fermentation. We achieve this by either using naturally acidic ingredients like lemons, berries, or vinegars, or by capitalizing on the natural production of acetic acid, citric acid, and lactic acid by microbes. In the south of Japan, where conditions are warmer and more prone to spoilage, *Aspergillus kawachii* became popular due to its ability to produce citric acid and lower the pH of its ferments. The high level of acidity is also why a fully developed vinegar will last forever.

MEASURING ACIDITY WITH PH

Throughout this book, I will refer to the pH of certain recipes. The pH, or potential of hydrogen, is a logarithmic scale of the level of acidity. Introduced by the Danish chemist Søren Peter Lauritz Sørensen in 1909, pH measures the potential difference in concentration between hydrogen ions and hydroxide ions to give us a valuable indication of acidity.

The scale goes from 0 to 14, with 7 representing neutrality, 0 being highly acidic, and 14 being highly alkaline. Water—at 77°F (25°C)—is often completely neutral, while an ingredient like lemon juice is between 2 and 3. However, every number on the pH scale indicates a change in value 10 times that of the previous number, meaning lemon juice is between 10,000 and 100,000 times more acidic than water. I use a pH meter to measure my ferments, but you can also use a color-changing indicator (pH paper).

It is important for safety to know the pH of your ferments, and, along with temperature, pH is one of the key influences on enzyme function.

PH AND ACIDITY SCALE

ACID TO NEUTRAL TO ALKALINE		PH VALUE	ACIDITY SCALE
	BATTERY ACID	0	1
	STOMACH ACID	1	0.1
	LEMON JUICE, LIME JUICE, AND MOST VINEGARS	2	0.01
	ORANGE JUICE, RHUBARB, AND RASPBERRIES	3	0.001
	TOMATOES, SOURDOUGH BREAD, AND HONEY	4	0.0001
	BANANAS, MAPLE SYRUP, ONIONS, AND SUGAR	5	0.00001
	MILK (+BUTTER), MUSHROOMS, PEAS, AND MELON	6	0.000001
	WATER	7	0.0000001
	EGGS AND SEAWATER	8	0.00000001
	BAKING SODA	9	0.000000001
	GREAT SALT LAKE (UTAH) AND MILK OF MAGNESIA	10	0.0000000001
	AMMONIA SOLUTION	11	0.00000000001
	SOAPY WATER	12	0.000000000001
	LYE WATER AND BLEACH	13	0.0000000000001
	DRAIN CLEANER	14	0.00000000000001

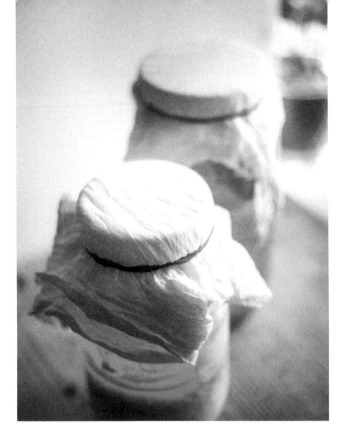

Breathable cloth lids for aerobic fermentation secured with elastic bands.

OXYGEN (AEROBIC VS. ANAEROBIC)

There are three types of microbes used in fermentation: those that require oxygen to thrive, those that don't, and those that can adapt to either condition. An example of the latter is lactic acid bacteria (LAB, see p.64), the first microorganism you'll be acquainted with in the recipes. It can survive with or without oxygen, happily converting sugar into lactic acid and producing carbon dioxide. However, another bacteria, acetic acid bacteria (AAB, see p.65), requires oxygen to feed on both sugar and alcohol. This is why an airlock is required when making alcohol to give yeast the opportunity to convert the fruit sugars into ethanol uninterrupted by the greedy AAB, which can outrun it. While yeast thrives in an oxygen-free environment, cracking open the airlock will give AAB the opportunity it needs to happily feed on the ethanol and convert it into acetic acid. This is why a bottle of wine left open will turn into vinegar without any intervention. And why wine can last forever within a sealed bottle. For the recipes, I will advise if they require aerobic or anaerobic fermentation (or if it doesn't matter).

INOCULATION

Inoculation is the controlled exposure of a food to friendly microbiology in order to ensure a ferment springs into action. In yogurt-making, we'll use a spoonful of tangy natural yogurt to set off a fresh batch of milk. Vinegar mothers and kombucha SCOBYs can outlive people and be used regularly for decades to inoculate the harvest of fruits and teas. As previously mentioned, we often use a technique called "backslopping" (see p.24) to inoculate a new ferment with a mature batch of microbes. This helps make sure the new ferment starts off on the right foot, with a healthy, active community of microbes we know work well. There are times when this technique yields better taste and texture, such as the fermented grains (see pp.112–113), which preserve a springy texture and better color thanks to the activity of the mature inoculation.

However, there are times when inoculation isn't desirable or necessary. Lacto fermentation (see p.66) will happen spontaneously given the right conditions, and, in such a ferment (known as wild fermentation), a lot of the flavor and joy of it comes from the concoction of wild microbes. At the other end of the spectrum, yeast and mold fermentation require us to push the odds in their favor more. There are wine yeasts and Aspergillus spores that are carefully selected for an exact set of reliable traits. Think about bread. Buy a sachet of baker's yeast, and you'll reliably produce the same loaf each and every time. Cultivate your own sourdough starter, and it will carry its own unique characteristics that are distinct from any other but will take more time and effort to care for. So, although inoculation can be an important tool at your disposal, equally important is knowing when it isn't needed.

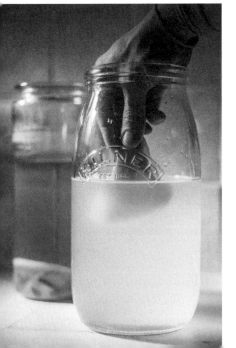

Vinegar mother and raw liquid vinegar being used to inoculate fresh mead.

Plums being weighed to
calculate how much salt
is required for lacto
fermentation.

FERMENTER'S PERCENTAGE

To offer flexibility for you to scale the recipes in this book to suit your needs, all recipes will be written as percentages. In fermentation, we take the total weight of the ingredients (including the weight of added water if a recipe requires it) as 100 percent and calculate everything else based on that. A recipe might call for 2 percent salt or 10 percent inoculation, meaning if the jar full of ingredients weighs 1kg, you'd need to add 20g salt or inoculate with 100g of a mature batch.

For the most part, I'll write the recipes as weightages, but I'll also include percentages where needed for ease of adaptation.

ACCURATE MEASUREMENTS

Throughout the recipes in this book, I have listed ingredients by weight in grams and kilograms. This makes following safe practice in fermentation much easier, as grams and kilograms are divisible by 10, so work nicely as a percentage. Pounds and ounces do not, and volume measurements (such as fluid ounces, milliliters, liters, and cups) often aren't as accurate as weights. Any recipes written with volume measurements are usually a result of dealing with larger, less accurate quantities or (in the case of alcohol fermentation) have other means of measurement, too, such as Brix and specific gravity (see p.117).

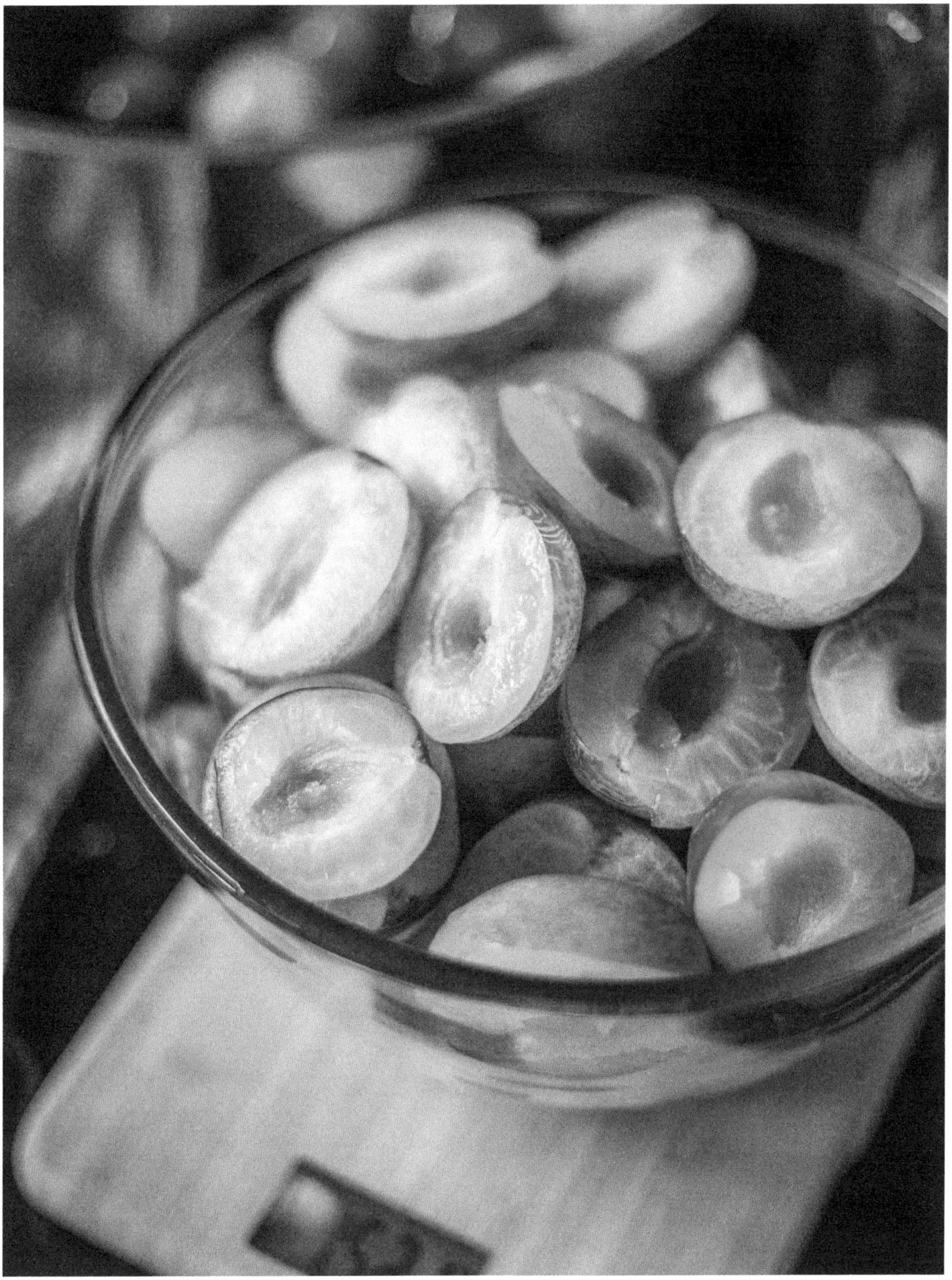

GETT*ING*
SET UP

It's time to make your own fermentation station. These can be as high tech or as simple as your needs and budget dictate. I'll go over everything I use, including the regular household kitchen equipment and appliances, up to the more niche investments you'll need to buy for an ideal setup.

To get started, all you'll need is a jar and salt. But to manage every recipe in this book, you'll need the following.

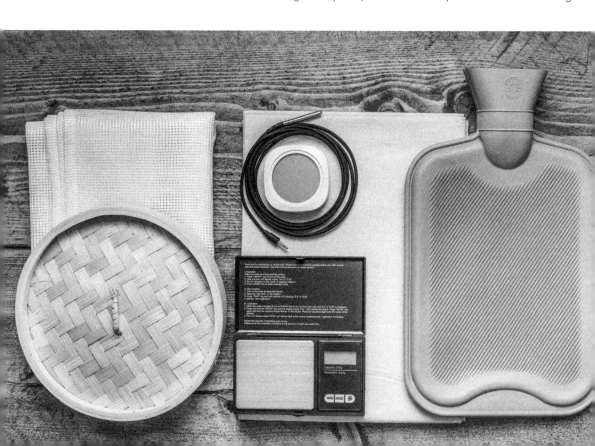

REGULAR HOUSEHOLD ITEMS

Most of the items below will already be in your kitchen and will be invaluable for your culinary adventures in fermenting.

- **Kettle** It's important you have access to boiling water in fermentation.
- **Dish towels** Most people have them, but you're going to need 6–7 or so set aside for fermentation. It's important that they're cotton, lint free, and clean.
- **Elastic bands or string** To secure breathable lids on jars.
- **Nonreactive utensils** These can be wood, silicone, or stainless steel. Serving spoons are the most useful. Some say metal is bad for microbes and will inhibit fermentation, but this is only true for reactive metals. This is why commercial kombucha is made in huge stainless-steel tanks without any issues.
- **Scales** For the most part, regular kitchen scales will do, but later in the book, you'll need to measure 0.1 of a gram, so if you're eager to make every recipe here, you'll need sensitive digital scales.
- **Hot-water bottle** Nothing fancy, no cover.
- **Baking sheet and wire rack** These need to be nonreactive material and the rack should fit within the sheet, leaving 5–6cm of sheet above it. My sheets are 23 × 31cm.
- **Multicooker** Possibly not that common in every country, a multicooker is the easiest and most affordable way to tackle some of the recipes in this book, from making amazake (see pp.176–179) and black garlic (see pp.102–103) to dehydrating and pasteurizing. I advise you to get a mini one—1.8-liter-capacity at most.

An assortment of basic kōji fermentation equipment. From left to right: a steaming cloth, steamer lid, temperature and humidity probe, scales, canvas, and a hot-water bottle.

VESSELS

Your ferments need a home to live in. We ourselves make perfectly comfortable homes for many microbes, but for the same reasons we do, a jar, ceramic crock, clay pot, glass bottle, demijohn, lunch box, or vacuum-sealed bag are also ideal. Anything that can create an inside and an outside can be used, even a bowl with a plate resting on top.

Your choice of vessel is up to you and depends on what you're making. Throughout this book, you'll see a range of different glass jars and some vacuum-sealed bags. I also use ceramic crocks, taking care not to use anything with a reactive glaze, but for the sake of demonstrating the recipes in this book, the transparency of glass works better. The issue with glass is UV light, which can help or hinder microbial growth. (UV is always damaging to microbes, but there are some ferments that are prone to kahm yeast, a harmless but unpleasant-tasting biofilm that can grow on the surface. There is some evidence that storing a ferment

DEMIJOHN

Also called Carboy, these vessels are characterized by their large bodies and narrow neck and opening.

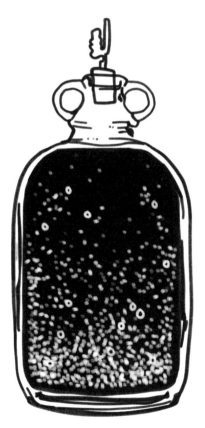

in direct sunlight can slow or halt the growth of such yeasts, but I cannot speak for the effectiveness of this technique, nor the impact on the rest of your ferment.) Some fermenters use colored glass vessels, as this protects the contents from UV, and often a windowsill is one of the naturally warmest places to leave your bubbling jar. I have a set of shelves that act as my fermentation station, but you could pick a cabinet or countertop, or anywhere that's not directly in sunlight but still warm: 64–86°F (18–30°C).

CROCK

Ceramic crocks are one of the oldest fermentation and preserving vessels.

Using a shallow moat of water around the rim, the crock lid allows gas to escape while protecting the food inside from pests and oxygen.

JAR

One of the most common choices for fermenters today, jars come in all shapes and sizes, ideal for any kitchen.

Microbes inside can build up pressure, so a jar requires "burping" daily at the beginning of fermentation.

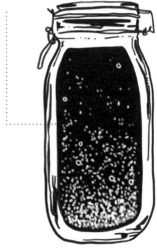

AIRLOCKS

BUBBLER AIRLOCKS
A one-piece tube that stops liquid from flowing backward into your ferment.

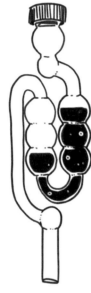

TWO-PIECE AIRLOCKS
A two-piece design that's easier to take apart and clean.

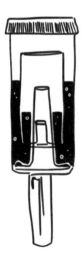

Hand-in-hand with the vessels you choose to ferment in are the types of lids and functionality of them. Some ferments require us to keep oxygen out but let carbon dioxide escape, and for large batches of very active fermentation, an airlock can make your life a lot easier. There are a few different types of airlocks, but the main ones come with pros and cons.

Bubbler airlocks These are the twisted tube designs you probably saw in your grandfather's home-brew demijohns. These are very low maintenance, as the water inside has a very slow evaporation rate; however, they can be troublesome to clean.

Two-piece airlocks These are lidded and cylindrical in design, which makes them far easier to clean between ferments, but I've found the water inside evaporates much more quickly. So bear in mind that you'll have to check them more frequently and top them up, or you run the risk of your wine turning into vinegar.

Makeshift airlocks So you don't want to buy an airlock, but you have lots of elastic bands lying around? Fasten one tightly around the clip of a regular jar (enough to hold the lid shut), but don't lock the clip. As pressure builds from the production of carbon dioxide, the elastic band will stretch, letting the gas escape, while keeping oxygen from getting in.

Water-sealed crocks This type of ceramic crock offers an ingenious solution from a time before plastic airlocks. The crock has an extra-deep rim, which acts as a moat to contain water. When the lid is placed on top, sitting within the water, the water forms a seal against the external atmosphere. As gas builds up, the lid is pushed up enough to allow bubbles to escape, but the air on the outside never manages to get back in. The best part about this design? It is built into the crock itself, so there are no additional parts to worry about—and it's easy to clean between batches. The downside: water can evaporate faster than you'd expect, and it can fill up with fruit flies if you're using fruit or berries.

STEAMERS

For the kōji recipes later in the book, it is important that you manage to steam your chosen substrate effectively. Here, I've added a breakdown of different steamers. There are many to choose from, each with its own benefits and drawbacks. If you have a steamer already, then that's perfect—don't go out and buy another. They all work, but for our needs, some are easier to work with than others. Alternatively, you can get away with a sieve over a saucepan of boiling water with a lid resting on top.

TYPES OF STEAMERS
Steaming is mainly important for making kōji, but there are many types of steamers.

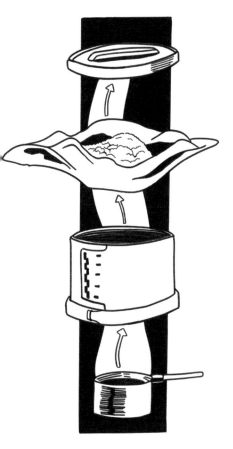

Bamboo steamers These are the most commonly accessible of the traditional steamers, but their open slats don't generate much steam pressure, so they tend to cook grains from the bottom up. A way around this is to open them up partway through cooking and turn the ingredients over, but the more they're handled, the more they will start to fall apart. You can purchase a metal steamer rack for it to sit on, which has holes instead of slats and will help generate more ideal conditions.

Wooden steamers These are much harder to track down and tend to be more expensive. The difference in their design is that they're often square; made from solid wood; and crucially, allow steam in via just one or two holes in the base. This generates pressure, forcing the steam deep into the rice or barley, creating a more even finish to the cooked grain.

Stainless-steel steamers These are hard-wearing and also generate steam pressure nicely, but have a tendency to collect condensed water in the base, oversaturating the lower layers of rice. This can be countered by rotating the grain partway through, but the last thing you want to do is open the lid too often and crash the temperature inside. Also, the less often you put your hands in a steamer, the lower your chances of burning yourself.

*WEI*GHTS

These come in all shapes and sizes, so make sure you get ones that are compatible with your chosen vessels. Glass tends to be made as a singular disk, while ceramic often comes in two halves, making them easier to insert. You can also use food-safe zip-lock plastic bags filled with spare grain or water as a weight; a small, clean jam jar filled with something heavy; or even a smooth stone. If using a stone, look for something nonporous—with no visible marking of heavy metals—that's been made completely smooth by erosion, then clean and sterilize it by boiling it.

WEIGHTS

One of the most important and useful pieces of equipment for vessel-based fermentation, as solid ingredients must be held below the surface of the brine.

Glass weights are one of the most simple and practical to use.

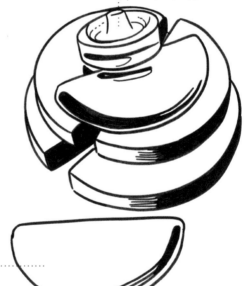

Ceramic weights often come in two halves, but unglazed ceramics can house microbes, so take care cleaning them.

PH METER

Pour a small amount of fermented liquid into a separate container and test the acidity with a pH meter.

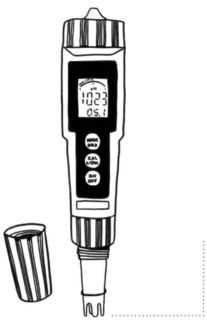

The sensor is located on the tip.

PH ME*TER*

As mentioned in the section on salt and acid (see pp.35–37), being able to monitor the pH of a ferment is very important for both safety and flavor. Both pH meters and indicator strips are readily available online and equally affordable. A pH meter requires calibration to make sure it remains accurate. This is done by preparing buffers (solutions that come with the pH meter in the form of sachets). Instructions may vary depending on the model, but most importantly, make sure the ferment is at the correct temperature, as this can affect the reading.

HYDROMETER

This ingenious device measures the relative density of liquids using buoyancy. This is important in fermentation, as it allows us to keep an eye on the gradual changes in liquids like beer and wine as dissolved sugars are replaced with alcohol, lowering the overall density of the liquid. Liquids like acid, brine, and milk have a high density (compared to water), while alcohol has a low density. This is measured in relative density, also called specific gravity.

HYDROMETER

Hydrometers use buoyancy to indicate the amount of dissolved solids in a liquid.

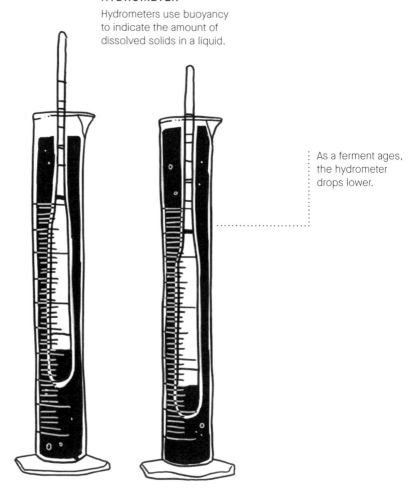

As a ferment ages, the hydrometer drops lower.

REFRACTOMETER

These measure the angle of
light passing through a liquid
to indicate the amount of
dissolved solids in the liquid.

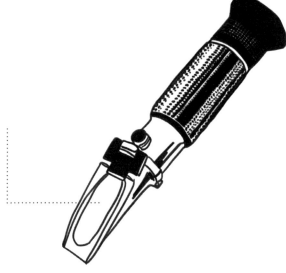

A single drop of liquid
is trapped against the
measuring prism.

REFRACTOME*TER*

This scientific-sounding instrument lets us easily check
the sugar levels in liquid, in a measurement called Brix
(see p.117). Later on, in the yeast recipes, it can be a
handy tool to measure the natural sugars in ingredients
and help calculate if you need to add more. These are
easy to find and quite affordable online.

HEAT*ING* MAT

While not essential, a simple, cheap heating mat from
a home-brew supply store or online is a useful way to
control ferments, especially over winter. Most of them
come with a probe to secure to the outside of the vessel
and a controller to set the exact temperature you
require. They are very useful for long-term ferments
like wine and mead that can span months and are a great
replacement for a hot-water bottle in the kōji-making
process (see pp.165–175).

CANVAS

A 1 × 1m piece of untreated canvas is perfect for kōji-making, as you'll need to wrap it up snugly in the initial 24 hours of growth. While dish towels might seem suitable for the job, a piece of canvas is ideal for insulating both temperature and humidity, the latter being paramount for healthy kōji.

INSULATED FOOD CARRIER BOX

INSULATED FOOD CARRIER

A great way to control the temperature of fermenting foods, especially sensitive ones like kōji.

This is another item for the ideal kōji setup, although you can certainly manage without it if you have an oven you won't need for 48 hours. I use a 46-liter-capacity carrier box because it's the ideal size for my home kōji needs. It is also easy to clean and store out of the way under a bed or on the top shelf of a closet when not in use. Later, in the mold section, I'll outline both oven-based kōji growing and insulated carrier box techniques, with the benefits and drawbacks. But I prefer the level of control with an insulated box.

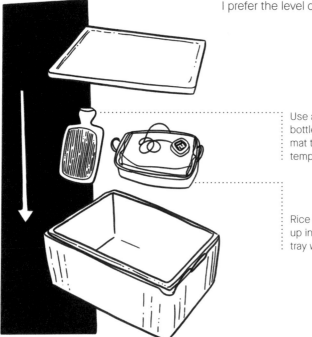

Use a hot-water bottle or heating mat to maintain temperature within.

Rice kōji wrapped up in a prepared tray with probe.

PROBE THERMOME*TER*

Essential for kōji fermentation, probe thermometers come in all shapes and sizes. Perfectly affordable and readily available online, look for one that monitors both temperature and humidity and ideally has Bluetooth or Wi-Fi connectivity so you can monitor your ferment without disturbing it.

VACUUM SEALER

Sous vide, cooking under vacuum, is a popular chef technique in restaurants, but even more useful in fermentation. While ingredients always run the risk of going wrong in a jar or crock, in a vacuum-sealed environment, the chances are reduced exponentially. The downside is plastic use; however, you can now get a hold of compostable bags, although they are more expensive. The cheaper design is a clamp sealer, but these struggle with liquids. Ideally, you'd need a chamber sealer, but these are larger—about the size of a microwave. It's worth noting, if you do make the investment, you can use a vacuum sealer for much more than fermentation, so weigh your options and, if you're thrifty, check out refurbished machines.

MULTICOO*KER*

If your kitchen has room for only one microwave-sized object, I'd opt for a multicooker any day of the week. Not only can you use them as a pressure cooker, rice cooker, small oven, grill, or even dehydrator, but they also have a "keep warm" function and a yogurt-making function, making them ideal for amazake (see pp.176–179), too. While they aren't the cheapest appliance out there (mine cost $315 [£249]), they certainly are the most versatile, and they're useful in ways the manufacturers probably didn't intend.

DEHYDRATOR

If you're into long-term preservation and want an option that doesn't turn everything into mush (we're looking at you, freezers), then a dehydrator is ideal. While you don't need it for any of the active fermentation in this book, it can be useful for capturing ingredients at the peak of their flavor and extending their ambient shelf life. It's also a great way to transform ingredients into crispy deliciousness or chewy treats, and who doesn't want that? The drawbacks are that they can be bulky and more of a financial investment, so explore all the recipes in this book before buying one, although the cost of running a dehydrator is outweighed by the shelf life and it's cheaper than running a freezer all year.

YOUR FERMENTATION STATION

LABELLING FERMENTS

It's usually good practice to label your ferments using masking tape and marker pen or food safety labels. I tend to include a start date, salt percentage, and name for a batch of whatever I'm making (for example: 26.09.21, 14%, yellow split peas and barley shoyu). Not all labels and tape come away cleanly afterwards, but using hot water can help loosen stubborn marks left on the glass.

This is a fancy name for a set of shelves, the size and shape of which depends on how deep you want to go down the fermentation rabbit hole and what kind of space you have in your house. Ideally, you want a room where the temperature is relatively constant, and in a position where it isn't blasted with sunlight all day. Mine is metal for ease of cleaning, with adjustable shelves, but you can use anything you like, from an old bookcase to a vacant kitchen cabinet. I store equipment on the bottom shelf; use the middle shelves for active ferments; and use the top shelves for long-term aging, such as wine, vinegar, miso, and shoyu (as these don't need monitoring as closely). It is important to keep on top of cleaning, especially when so many ferments have fabric lids. Dust and debris from the shelves above can settle and risk contamination on breathable ferments, so make sure you clean the station once a month with a degreaser.

Shelving (out of direct sunlight) stores an assortment of fermented, preserved, and dried ingredients.

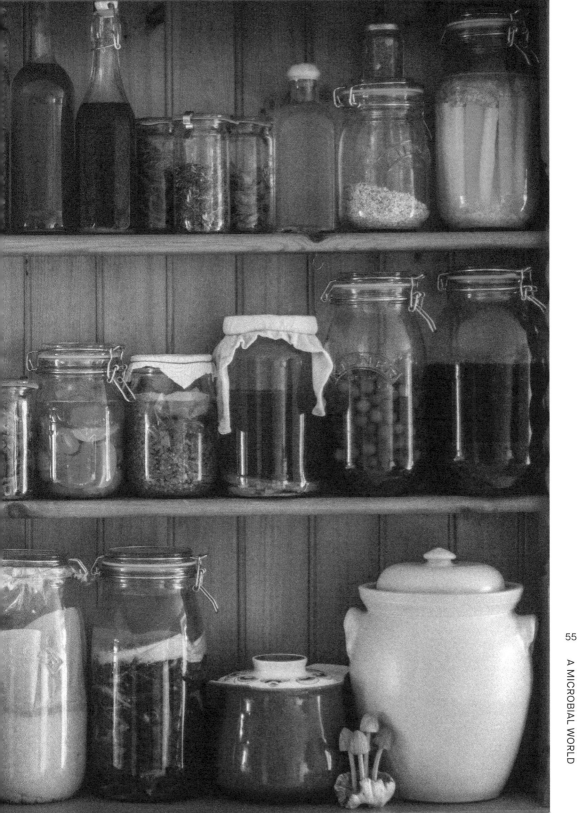

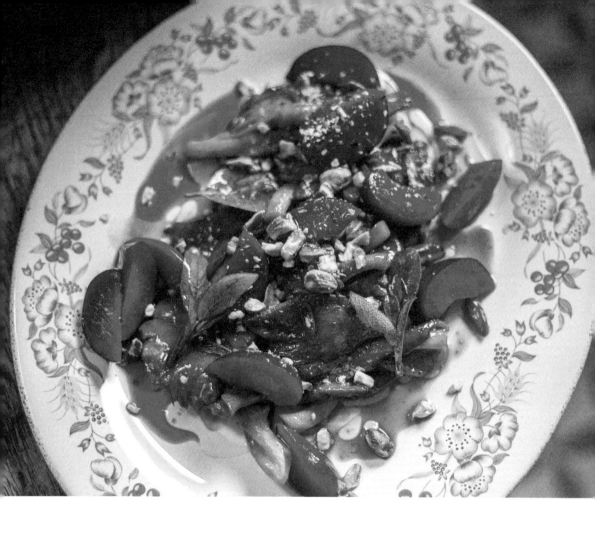

COOKING WITH
FERMENTED
FOODS

Fermented lacto plums
with braised mushrooms,
pistachio, and sage.

Although the main focus of this book is a journey through
the many types of fermentation, along the way, I have also
included my favorite ways to use fermented ingredients in
everyday meals. My approach to creating dishes that make
the most of fermented foods has three considerations at its
heart: taste, aroma, and texture.

TASTE

Broadly speaking, fermented foods fall into these main
flavors: acidic, umami, and salty. They're also often very
powerful flavors, far too strong to eat as they are. This
is where pairing comes into play. By pairing a potent
ferment with a counter flavor that balances its dominant
characteristics, we're able to detect and enjoy the range
of subtle flavors that were previously overpowered. For
example, pairing miso with sweet flavors (like squash,
pumpkin, or apple) or with nutty flavors (like hazelnut,
sesame, or brown butter) can diminish its funky saltiness,
giving you access to its fruity, earthy, sometimes even
buttery sweet notes.

The reverse is also true. You can use a small amount
of a strong fermented ingredient to balance or enhance
other ingredients. For example, the saltiness of a shoyu or
garum balances bitter ingredients like chicory and broccoli.
The key is knowing how these main flavors interact, then
looking for ways to combine them. Why not char the
chicory for some additional smokiness, then brush it with
shoyu? Add a squeeze of fresh orange juice to offer clarity
and freshness, simultaneously balancing the bitterness
further while also giving the shoyu's umami a boost.
Or better yet, add the orange to the pan with the chicory
and use the heat to draw out fragrant oils from the skin.

Overleaf is my go-to flavor diagram, highlighting the
main relationships between these flavors. I encourage you
to play. Explore your ferments and see what works for you.
And the next time you're eating out, pay close attention to
the construction of each dish. You never know when you
might discover a whole new pairing.

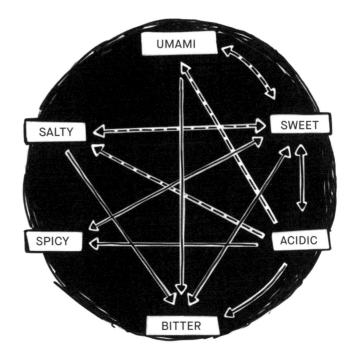

FLAVOR INTERACTIONS

The solid-line arrows indicate flavors that balance the other; dotted arrows signify those that enhance. Two-way arrows show flavors that are mutually balancing or enhancing.

These flavor interactions are in part why kimchi works so well. It is acidic, spicy, salty, and bitter. Both the saltiness and acidity balance the bitterness of cabbage, and the acidity enhances the spice. Understanding the interactions between flavors is key to using the bold flavors produced by fermentation in your cooking.

FAT

Fat also gets an honorary mention as a flavor, although often overlooked. Interestingly, this could be due to a limited vocabulary in the description of fat-related flavors, highlighting the importance of language around food. Words offer a handle on thoughts and a useful label that can act, in equal part, as an entry point and a means to communicate. Think of all the ways the flavors of wine are described, or coffee. Vocabulary is an important factor in both describing and understanding flavor. Besides fat's role in richness and a range of textures, it can offer fermented ingredients a complementary pairing with acidic, punchy, and umami flavors. Fat is also celebrated in the culinary world for its greatly significant ability to capture aroma, which fermented foods are packed full of, leading us neatly onto the next section.

AROMA

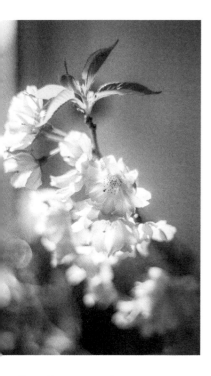

Cherry blossom, one of many seasonal aromatic ingredients we can capture using fermentation.

AROMA, EMOTION, AND MEMORIES

Aroma, almost more than anything else, can stimulate emotions and memories. This happens because the parts of the brain responsible for identifying odors are also responsible for memory and emotion. This is why the scent of a long-forgotten herb can send you crashing back to your childhood, standing in your grandmother's kitchen, salivating over a pie you've not had for 30 years.

If there are seven main flavors, why do we have so many words describing food? Meaty, cheesy, mossy, earthy, buttery, nutty, fruity, fishy ... the list is vast. If apples are sweet, but so are pears, how can we tell them apart by taste alone? And why is it that coffee can be described as dark chocolate, blueberry, orange blossom, or marzipan? Well, this is thanks to your nose. Your sense of smell is many times more sensitive than the flavors detected by your tongue. The olfactory system can detect over a trillion unique odors by distinguishing the different bonds between molecules that float your way. This happens as the food releases aroma compounds into the air on its way to your mouth and via retronasal olfaction, creating flavor from the perception of aroma molecules that drift up the nasal passage as you eat.

Ingredients also have aromas in common. Take vanilla, which is 1–2 percent vanillin, a chemical compound we can detect with our sense of smell. It is also found in oak and naturally extracted when alcohol is aged in oak barrels, giving us vanilla notes in whisky. The same is true for pairing unrelated ingredients, such as watercress and goat cheese, which have completely different flavors but share a minerality (see *The Flavour Thesaurus* by Niki Segnit for more). You can also find this within the signatures of fermented foods thanks to the microbes responsible for them. For example, both the nukadoko (see p.211) and Parmesan cheese contain butyric acid bacteria, giving them both the same characteristic odor.

Aroma compounds are highly sensitive to heat, so cooking will destroy some and release others. The same is true for the opposite, and chilling a fermented ingredient will sometimes diminish its funkiness and pave the way for its more pleasant, less dominant characteristics. For example, the pea and spelt shoyu (see pp.202–207), when exposed to the heat of a broth once it's been poured into a serving bowl, unlocks notes of brioche. But if added into the hot oil of a frying pan, it loses these instantly and develops deep, almost cheesy umami.

TEXT*URE*

Two words come to mind most in describing the textures of fermented ingredients: crunchy and soft. There are, of course, liquids, too, but these are a step away from texture and move into the realm of mouthfeel. Apparently, the word "crispy" has the biggest selling power in all of food marketing. That's how important texture is.

There are a whole host of fermented foods that are prized for their crunch, and in fact, you can prepare the ingredients ahead of time specifically to improve this characteristic. Leaving veggies chunky for a kimchi or lacto ferment will give a wonderful crunch, while grating or chopping them finely will reduce this. Crunch is prized not just for the satisfaction of an audible snap as you bite it, but also because it kicks up aroma as you chew, acting as a mini flavor catapult in your mouth, sending aromatic compounds up your nasal passage. At the other end of the spectrum, we have soft ferments like miso, lacto tomatoes (which can even be fizzy), and lacto berries. These ferments are easily incorporated into broths and sauces, where combining with the fat of a butter or oil will carry their aroma throughout a dish.

Quick pickled garlic, radish, cucumber, and red pepper using shio kōji, which seasons and softens the ingredients while preserving a satisfying crunch.

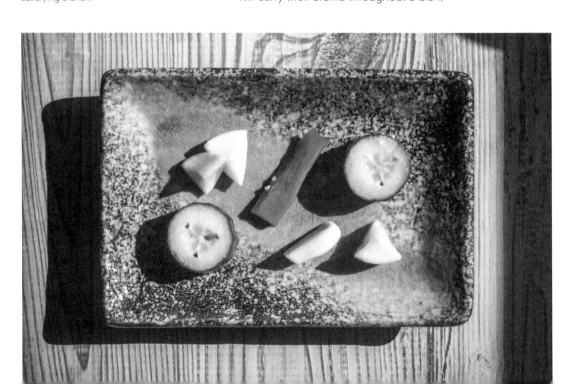

If you wish to alter the texture of fermented foods, consider cooking crunchy ingredients to soften them or drying them to make them crispy. You can even turn them into powders and smuggle them into sauces, pasta, or bread doughs. For liquids, try reducing them over a low heat to thicken them and concentrate their flavor.

While many people understand the importance of texture, it's often an overlooked part of a meal compared to flavor and smell, but when used cleverly or really perfected, it can elevate an eating experience.

TEMPERATURE

Temperature can unlock new dimensions within fermented ingredients, such as turning soured cabbage into charred, cheesy flavor bombs. A lot of people eat fermented foods for the living microbes, which doesn't work if you plan to cook them. But the real powerhouses here are enzymes. In the same way that we humans have hugely benefited from the production of penicillin from mold, the nutritional value of fermented foods—thanks to the enzymes of microbes—goes through the roof. Enzymes are what make a humble boiled bean become a fruity, umami-rich miso, and similar is true for acids and their breakdown of complex molecules.

However, enzymes aren't only sensitive to temperature, they also denature when exposed to a strong acidic environment (such as your stomach). So all the benefits have to take place before we eat them.

This means that some fermented foods, such as shoyu (see p.202) and miso (see p.191), shouldn't be cooked for too long or too hot, as it will destroy their more complex, fragrant qualities, while others can be subjected to all sorts of cooking. Emulsifying lacto tomato brine (see p.68) into a butter makes a fruity, deeply savory glaze, and the legendary flavors of a kimchi grilled cheese (see p.95) are celebrated far and wide. The same is true for the opposite. Chilling a kombucha, beer, or lacto ferment can diminish overpowering characteristics in favor of more subtle, refreshing notes. So don't be afraid to explore the world of cooking with your fermented foods as an additional step.

The smallest of our hungry friends, bacteria's ability to multiply as it feeds on the natural sugars present in fruits, vegetables, and mushrooms makes it the perfect choice for those who are starting their fermenting journey. There are countless varieties of these single-celled organisms found in every known environment.

BACTERIA

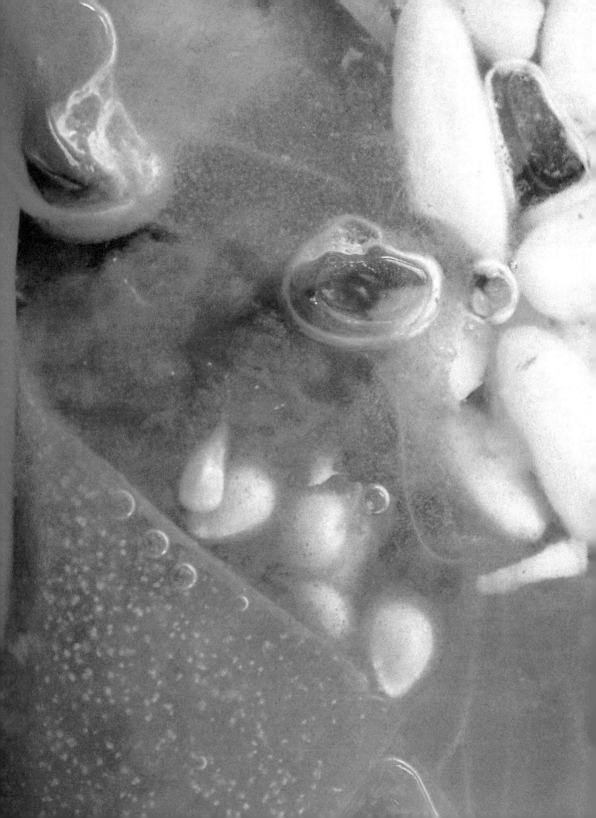

INTRODUCING BACTERIA

While some bacteria produce toxins, the two that we will focus on in this book produce acid, specifically lactic acid (the very same that your muscles generate when exercising) and acetic acid (which gives vinegar its tart, lip-smacking liveliness).

LACTIC ACID BACTERIA (LAB)

Kimchi, sauerkraut, pickles, and yogurt are all products of lactic acid bacteria (LAB). They are commonly found on the skins of all things with skin, from plants to people, and produce a distinct and delicious sourness. Quick acting, salt tolerant, and ideally suited to aerobic and anaerobic fermentation (they thrive with or without oxygen), these bacteria naturally protect themselves and the ingredients they ferment by producing lactic acid, creating an environment that is inhospitable to many pathogens.

LACTIC ACID BACTERIA

A single LAB cell and the smallest microbe in our fermentation flock, capable of souring foods faster than almost any other microbe.

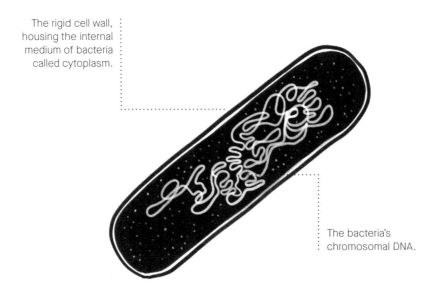

The rigid cell wall, housing the internal medium of bacteria called cytoplasm.

The bacteria's chromosomal DNA.

ACETIC ACID BACTERIA

The bacteria responsible for turning wine into vinegar.

The growth of AAB colonies within a fermenting medium, reaching up to 4.5μm in length.

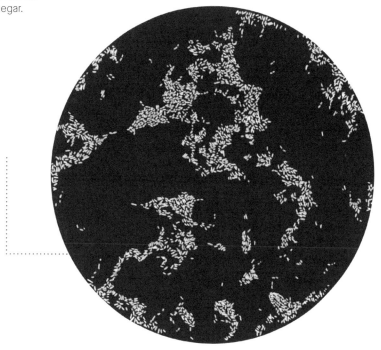

ACETIC ACID BACTERIA (AAB)

While we're introducing bacteria, I'll introduce you to the other acid-producing bacteria, acetic acid bacteria (AAB). AAB often appears in response to yeast activity and therefore will be found within the Yeast chapter of this book. If you're a fan of kombucha and the world of vinegars, then you've experienced the delicious sourness of AAB. These bacteria are celebrated for their ability to oxidize ethanol to acetic acid, which is released into the fermentative medium. Not only are they highly resistant to acidic environments, but they're also characterized by their production of extracellular polymers, such as bacteria cellulose (the jellyfish-looking rafts that float around in jars), which offer a range of applications, from food additives to wound dressings.

LACTO FERMENTAT*ION*

You can lacto ferment any vegetable, fruit, berry, or mushroom with a simple rule: 2 percent salt. Most varieties of lactic acid bacteria can tolerate up to 6.5 percent salt, which, in some cases, can be used to turn ingredients into salty caper alternatives. The increased amount of salt also has different effects on the ingredients you ferment, so have fun and explore. I tend to stick with my golden rule of 2 percent, partially because of flavor and partially because of health.

For ingredients like tomatoes, peaches, and cabbages, adding the salt is sufficient to draw out enough moisture from the ingredients themselves and make the fermenting brine. Other ingredients require the addition of water (the weight of which must be taken into consideration when calculating the amount of salt needed). Some ingredients, such as cranberries, benefit from being cut or lightly crushed before fermentation, as their skins form a tough barrier for bacteria. And some, such as mushrooms, require steaming to preserve their texture (which means you will need to add other raw ingredients, such as garlic, ginger, or radish, to act as an inoculant).

But still, the guiding principle remains. Your first step into the most accessible and simple form of fermentation is simply salt (dissolved in enough liquid to submerge the ingredients) in an airtight container. Within this rule, you can experiment to your heart's content and never run out of new discoveries. The following recipes in this chapter are some of my favorite and most interesting ways to ferment within this niche.

TWO METHODS FOR LACTO FERMENTATION

Lacto fermentation can be done in one of two ways. The first is in a glass jar or ceramic crock, held down with weights. The second is in a vacuum-sealed bag. There are pros and cons to each, which apply to all lacto-fermented ingredients. A crock or jar can be fitted with an airlock, allowing the carbon dioxide to escape and essentially making a ferment that takes care of itself.

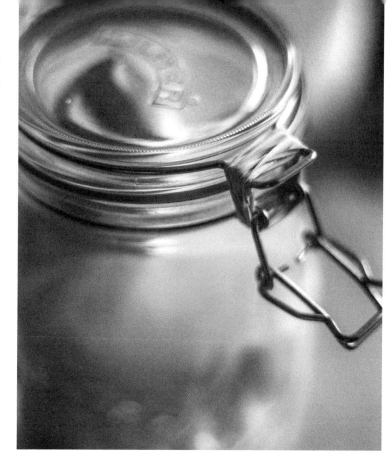

Using an elastic band to make a jar that releases carbon dioxide automatically.

MAKESHIFT AIRLOCKS AND "BURPING"

If you don't have an airlock, you can "burp" the jar daily by opening the lid to release the carbon dioxide. Alternatively (if going away or feeling lazy), secure the clip of the jar with an elastic band tightly enough to hold it down. As the pressure builds, the lid will lift enough to let some carbon dioxide out. To "burp" a vacuum bag, cut off a corner, gently squeeze it to release some carbon dioxide, then reseal.

A vacuum-sealed ferment will balloon with gas and requires burping (see left). Depending on the strength of your bag and your punctuality, a day too long may result in a messy pop. The downside to jar fermentation is you have to apply weight to the top, crushing the ingredients a little. If there isn't enough weight to submerge the ingredients below the level of the liquid, then there's a very real chance they will spoil and mold.

On the other hand, in a vacuum bag, the ingredients can roll around freely, retain their original splendor, and have virtually no risk of spoilage. Jars are also much more cumbersome to store when not in use, while vacuum sealers can be quite compact. But a jar is far less of a financial investment up front and reusable indefinitely if taken care of.

Lacto-fermented tomatoes, fully aged, make an incredible pan con tomate, salad, or gazpacho.

EQUIPMENT

1.5-liter glass jar or crock

glass or ceramic weight (roughly half the weight of the ingredients)

airlock or elastic band (optional)

or

vacuum bag

INGREDIENTS

1kg tomatoes

20g fine sea salt (2%)

Lacto tomatoes are delicious. They trick your brain into thinking you are tasting cooked tomatoes. Deeply umami and acidic, this recipe offers two finished ingredients that can elevate your home cooking. The tomato water (that becomes the fermenting brine) is deeply savory and complements soft cheeses, as well as being great in dressings, sauces, and glazes. The tomatoes themselves can be cooked into stews, turned into a salsa, served as bruschetta, or blended and topped with fresh cucumber and a peppery olive oil to make a supercharged gazpacho.

Sometimes lacto tomatoes can get fizzy and taste alcoholic. This isn't a bad thing and is most likely the work of a yeast called *Brettanomyces* or saison yeast. Commonly used for sour beer, when exposed to anaerobic conditions, *Brettanomyces* metabolizes sugar into ethanol. If this happens, you didn't do anything wrong; it was most likely already living on the skin of your tomatoes. If you don't like the fizz or flavor, cooking the fermented tomatoes removes it. Avoid it up front by fermenting tomatoes in a 2 percent saltwater solution instead of their juice.

LACTO TOMATOES

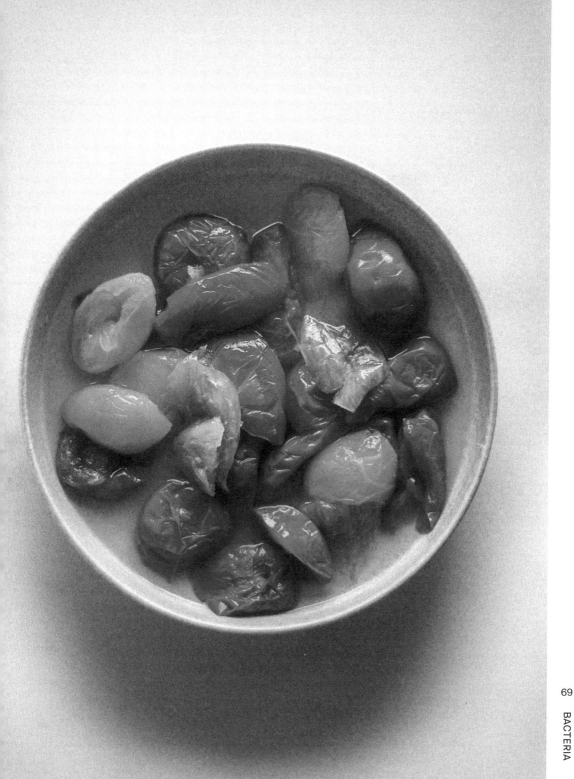

*USI*NG A JAR OR *CROCK*

1. Begin by washing and chopping the tomatoes. If using a selection of different varieties, leave small tomatoes whole, chop medium-sized tomatoes in half, and chop large tomatoes into quarters. This will increase the surface area and help you pack them into the jar.

2. In a bowl, mix the tomatoes and salt and pour it all into the jar. Make sure to get all the salt from the sides of the bowl. Place the weight on top.

3. Add an airlock and close the lid securely, making sure it's airtight, or use an elastic band around the clip (see p.67). Alternatively, you will need to burp it daily (see p.67).

4. Store at 68–86°F (20–30°C) on a shelf of your fermentation station for 5–7 days. By day 3, the salt should have drawn out enough liquid to completely cover the tomatoes. If not, you need to apply extra weight. Any ingredient that isn't submerged by brine will spoil.

5. Start tasting after 5 days, and once the tomatoes have reached your desired flavor, store in a fridge in an airtight container. The lacto tomatoes will last for a month in the fridge but will continue to ferment at a slower rate.

●

FERMENTER'S NOTE

This recipe in particular seems prone to kahm yeast when using in a jar. Turn to the section on kahm yeast in troubleshooting (see p.216) for how to counter this.

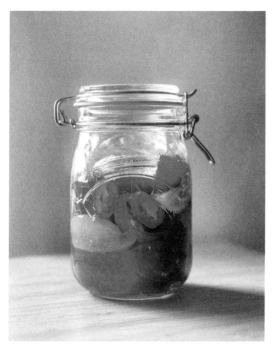

Day 1.

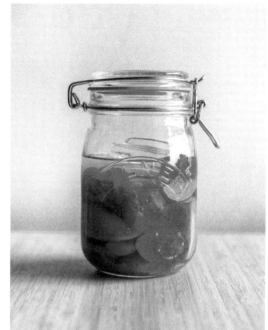

Day 3.

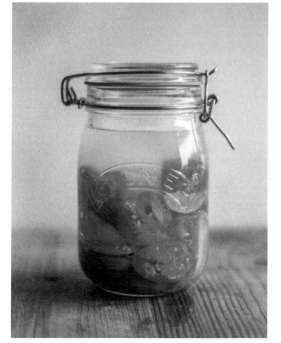

Day 7.

●

FERMENTER'S NOTE

If you don't have a glass or ceramic weight, you can use a food-safe bag filled with spare grain or water.

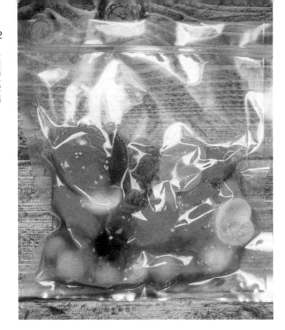
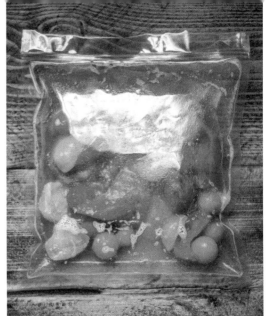

Top left Day 3.
Above Day 7.

USING A
VACUUM BAG

1. Begin by washing and chopping the tomatoes. If using a selection of different varieties, leave small tomatoes whole, chop medium-sized tomatoes in half, and chop large tomatoes into quarters. This will increase the surface area and help you pack them into the bag.

2. Put the chopped tomatoes into the vacuum bag so that they fit comfortably. Do not overfill the bag, as you will struggle to seal it later when liquid is released. Add the salt and give the ingredients a shake to distribute it evenly before vacuum sealing.

3. Store at 68–86°F (20–30°C) for 5–7 days on a shelf in your fermentation station. After day 2–3, keep a close eye on the bag, as the build-up of carbon dioxide will cause it to balloon; you may need to burp it (see p.67).

4. Once the ferment reaches your desired flavor, store the sealed bag in the fridge for up to a month, where it will continue to ferment but more slowly.

COOKING
WITH FERMENTS

TOMATO STEW

Cook lacto tomatoes and their brine with a mix of peppers, eggplants, fresh tomatoes, sweet potatoes, zucchini, thyme, and basil, then top with some homemade pesto.

TOMATO, SPINACH, AND MOZZARELLA SALAD

Combine lacto tomatoes with wilted spinach, chunks of mozzarella, fresh basil leaves, black pepper, and a good drizzle of olive oil.

GAZPACHO

Blend half lacto tomatoes and half fresh tomatoes with a clove of garlic, then top with a drizzle of peppery olive oil and some finely diced cucumber.

SALSA ROJA

Blend lacto tomatoes with some charred onion, chili, garlic, and lime juice.

PAN CON TOMATE

Rub garlic and lacto tomatoes into freshly toasted sourdough, then top with hard cheese.

SALAD DRESSING

Infuse the lacto tomato brine with herbs of your choice and mix with olive oil.

UMAMI GLAZE

Add the lacto tomato brine to ingredients such as mushrooms, whitefish, and sautéed vegetables cooking in a hot pan with butter.

UMAMI SEASONING

Dry in a dehydrator for 10 hours at 135°F (57°C) until bone dry, then blend.

PICKLING
WITH LACTO
BRINE

You can use leftover brine from ferments like lacto tomatoes or lacto berries (see pp.82–83) to create a vibrant and crunchy side dish, packed full of acidity and living microbes. Simply put julienned carrot, finely sliced red onion and radish, and trimmed green beans in a sealable lunch box or jar and add lacto brine to cover. Fasten the lid in place and put to the side for a minimum of 30 minutes or up to 24 hours. Eat as a side dish to a main dish, a crunchy addition to fresh salads and broths, or a great sandwich filler.

LACTO CAULIFLOWER

A potent-smelling ferment that becomes delicate and complex after two weeks, this recipe demonstrates how to ferment ingredients that don't produce enough moisture to make their own brine. Deliciously crunchy and sour, it can be eaten raw or charred; paired with mild, creamy cheeses; or ground into cauliflower rice. It's best done in a jar instead of a bag due to the size of the florets and quantity of liquid.

EQUIPMENT

2-liter jar

glass or ceramic weight

airlock or elastic band (optional)

INGREDIENTS

2 garlic cloves

1 cauliflower

salt (2%)

1. Peel the garlic and remove the outer leaves from the cauliflower. Cut the cauliflower into individual florets and give them a rinse under cold running water.

2. Tare scales to the weight of the jar and add the cauliflower and garlic. Fill with enough cold water to cover the ingredients, then take note of the combined weight of everything in the jar. Multiply this by 0.02 to calculate the grams of salt required. Add the salt, then close the lid and shake until all the salt is dissolved.

3. Open up the jar again and insert a weight to keep the ingredients from floating. Wipe the top down with a clean kitchen towel. Add an airlock and close the lid securely, making sure it's airtight, or use an elastic band around the clip (see p.67). Alternatively, you will need to burp it daily (see p.67).

4. Leave somewhere warm (around 70°F/21°C) for the next 1–2 weeks, then store for up to 2 months in the fridge.

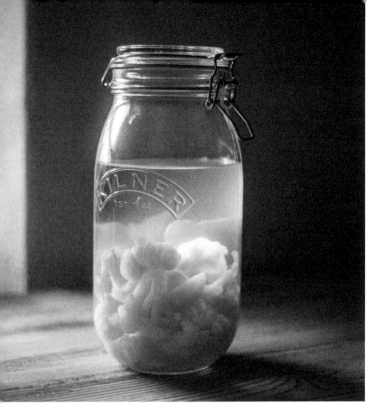

After day 7, the liquid turns clear again as the flavor mellows.

COOKING WITH FERMENTS

CAULIFLOWER, EMMENTAL, AND WILD GARLIC FLOWERS

Place lacto cauliflower pieces flat-side up on a baking sheet, top with a slice of Emmental cheese, and grill for 2 minutes until the cheese melts. Top with some wild garlic flowers and young mustard leaves.

FERMENTED CAULIFLOWER RICE

Crush the lacto cauliflower into a fermented cauliflower rice to liven up salads and side dishes, or blend into dips and sauces for a salty, lively kick.

LACTO CAULIFLOWER VARIATIONS

There are plenty of ways you can adapt this recipe once you've got the hang of it, simply by infusing it with extra flavorings or adding extra vegetables into the mix.

INFUSING LACTO CAULIFLOWER

If you've made this recipe before and want to mix things up, try infusing it with juniper, caraway, or other alliums (such as leeks, shallots, or garlic scapes).

USING UP LEFTOVERS

You can also use this recipe to turn waste scraps into delicious crunchy pickles by saving your kale and broccoli stems, diced up, and adding them in, too.

Right Plums on day 1 of fermentation, with a sealed bag of water as a weight.
Below A fresh plum beside a fermented plum, both halved.

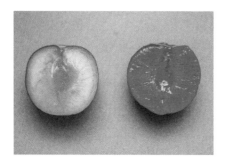

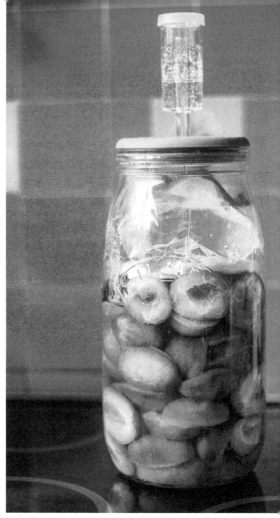

LACTO STONE FRUIT

Right Plums on day 1 of fermentation, with a sealed bag of water as a weight.
Below A fresh plum beside a fermented plum, both halved.

● **FERMENTER'S NOTE**

Reserve the brine, as this is a delicious, sour, salty juice that's been transformed into a wonderful marinade similar to the Japanese ume su, a tangy, salty-vinegar-like product made from plums. In small amounts, this brine can transform even dull black coffee into something elegant, smooth, and fruity.

Lacto peaches, plums, and nectarines are tart, sweet, and fragrant. Their skins are deeply sour and can be removed and dehydrated postfermentation and enjoyed as a seasoning that complements creamy flavors and seafood. The flesh infuses with a subtle ginger and smoky aroma that promotes their pairing in both savory and sweet uses. Smoked salt complements the fruit well, but normal sea salt can be used instead. You can make these ferments without any additional ingredients besides salt, but I wanted to use them as an example of a simple simultaneous fermentation and infusion, which is why I used ginger, too. For detailed instructions, follow the recipe for lacto tomatoes (see p.68).

EQUIPMENT

1.5-liter glass jar or crock

glass or ceramic weight

airlock or elastic band (optional)

or

vacuum bag

INGREDIENTS

1kg plums, peaches, or nectarines

21g smoked sea salt (2%)

10g ginger root, halved

1. For the best results, use ripe but not overly soft fruit. Halve the fruit and remove the stones. Add to the jar and mix in the smoked salt. Add the ginger and apply the weight. Alternatively, use a vacuum bag (see p.72).

2. Add an airlock and close the lid securely, making sure it's airtight, or use an elastic band around the clip (see p.67). Alternatively, you will need to burp it daily (see p.67).

3. By day 5–7, the fruit will be pleasantly sour and fragrant. If you want to preserve more texture, catch them at this stage. If you want a fruity, cidery flavor, age for another 3–4 days, but note that the flesh will start to break down.

4. Once fermented, they can be dehydrated and stored at room temperature in an airtight jar. To do so, remove the skin and dry the flesh separately at 140°F (60°C) for 10 hours. Or they will last 4 months in a fridge in an airtight container (packed in their brine).

In a lot of ferments that produce their own liquid, the leftover brine is a potent culinary product worth bottling.

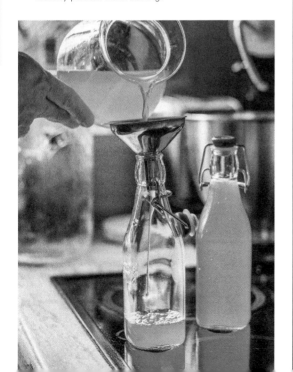

COOKING WITH FERMENTS

BRAISED MUSHROOMS WITH LACTO STONE FRUIT

Cook oyster mushrooms in a large frying pan with butter or oil and garlic, then add ale and a splash of Worcestershire sauce (or vegetarian or vegan alternative) and cook until syrupy. Serve topped with fermented stone fruit, some crushed pistachios, and a drizzle of the lacto brine.

GRILLED JUMBO SHRIMP WITH LACTO STONE FRUIT

Over the embers of a grill, cook seasoned jumbo shrimp for 3 minutes on each side and an extra 2 minutes on their backs. Mix chopped garlic in oil or melted butter, with a good glug of lacto stone fruit brine. Keep the sauce warm on the side of the grill and baste the jumbo shrimp throughout cooking. The fat will drop down and make fire, but this is fine. Eat right away.

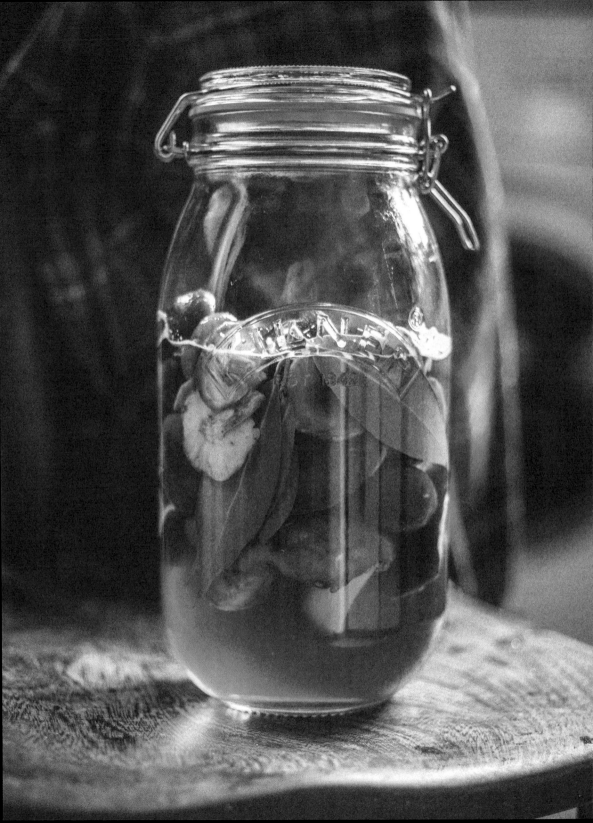

LACTO *SHIITAKE* IN ASSAM

EQUIPMENT

2-liter jar

glass or ceramic weight

airlock or elastic band (optional)

or

vacuum bag

INGREDIENTS

1.5kg water

1 Assam tea bag

45g sea salt (2%)

750g shiitake mushrooms

2 fresh bay leaves

1 tbsp shoyu (see pp.202–207) or light soy sauce

10g ginger root, halved

1 garlic clove

This ferment embraces the bold, tannic bitterness of Assam tea, balanced with the sour lacto goodness of mushroom depth. The first step is to steam the mushrooms, as this helps preserve their texture during fermentation. You can ferment mushrooms raw and they'll sometimes turn into a mildly alcoholic paste, which can be dehydrated and stored as a powder for up to a year. This recipe also introduces the idea of fermenting in different infusions. This works nicely for tea, but also for herbs and spices. As we're adding water instead of drawing it out from the ingredients, this will have to be taken into account when calculating the salt: the water, mushrooms, ginger, and garlic make up the "100 percent" from which the 2 percent salt has to be calculated.

Fermenting shiitake with bay, Assam, and shoyu unlocks mushroomy flavors while infusing with additional flavors.

1. Boil 500g water and add the tea to infuse for 5 minutes. Remove the tea bag and add the salt. Stir to dissolve the salt, and top it up with the remaining water to cool it down.

2. Remove any dirt or damaged parts from the mushrooms and place them in a steamer set above a pan of boiling water. Steam for 5–10 minutes.

3. Add the mushrooms to the jar, along with the tea, bay leaves, and shoyu. Make sure the liquid is below 95°F (35°C), then add the ginger and garlic. Apply a weight to hold the ingredients below the surface of the liquid. Alternatively, use the vacuum bag method (see p.72).

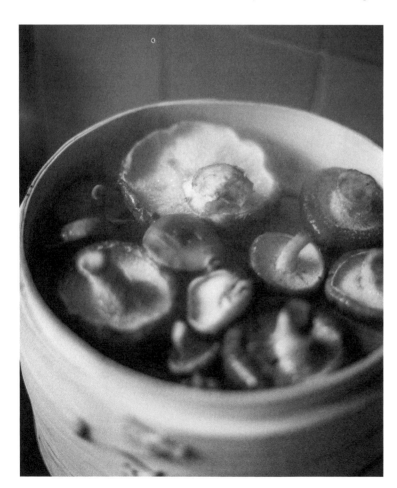

Steaming raw mushrooms helps retain their texture during fermentation.

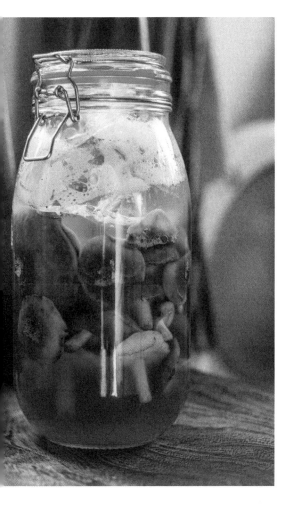

4. Add an airlock and close the lid securely, making sure it's airtight, or use an elastic band around the clip (see p.67). Alternatively, you will need to burp it daily (see p.67).

5. After 7 days, the mushrooms should have softened and soured, but you can continue to ferment them for another 7 days (14 in total) for an extra boost. After this point, store in the brine for up to 2 months in the fridge.

Day 7, fermented shiitake mushrooms in Assam.

COOKING WITH FERMENTS

DEHYDRATED LACTO SHIITAKE

Once fully fermented, dry the mushrooms in a dehydrator at 122°F (50°C) for 8–10 hours and store in an airtight container in a cabinet. Alternatively, blend the mushrooms with some of the fermented assam tea and dehydrate the paste, then blend again into a powder. This mushroomy, tannic powder is delicious mixed into cooked rice, pastry, and pasta dough or used as a spice seasoning.

PHYLLO, CABBAGE, AND LACTO SHIITAKE

Mix diced fermented shiitake with shredded savoy cabbage, grated ginger, crushed garlic, toasted sesame oil, and Worcestershire sauce (or vegan alternative). Wrap in phyllo pastry, brush with sunflower oil, and bake at 400°F (200°C) for 35 minutes.

LACTO
BERRIES

Lacto fermentation is a wonderful way to preserve berries and currants over the year. It's definitely worth mentioning that this ferment is nicest with a mild-tasting salt, such as Flor de Sal. However, for the opposite effect, you can increase the amount of salt to 6 percent, which turns the berries into a caperlike fruity alternative. Once made, every characteristic of fruity deliciousness is amplified, meaning you won't need much in other recipes to make a big impact.

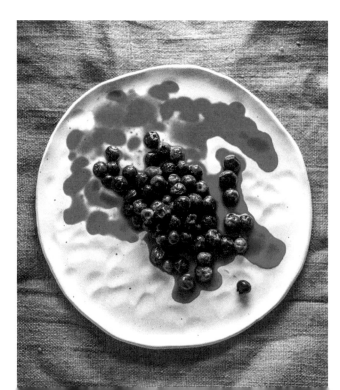

Fermented lacto berries on a plate.

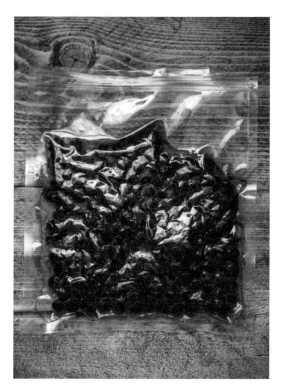

Day 3, fermenting
blueberries in vacuum.

COOKING WITH FERMENTS

SMOOTHIES
Add a small amount of lacto berries to smoothies.

BREAKFASTS
Use to top your breakfast (especially good with rye oatmeal).

CASSEROLES
Add to savory casseroles, where the fruity, salty, tannic qualities really shine.

SAUCES AND DIPS
Add a dash of fermented berry brine as a secret ingredient in sauces and dips.

FREEZE-DRIED BERRY POWDER
Collect the leftover brine and freeze-dry it into a salty berry powder that's perfect for dusting on rice pudding or ice cream.

COFFEE
Add a very small amount of berry brine to black coffee for a fragrant burst and smoother-tasting beverage.

EQUIPMENT
500ml jar

glass or ceramic
  weight

airlock or elastic
  band (optional)

or

vacuum bag

INGREDIENTS
150g berries

3g salt (2%)

1. Inspect the berries for damage or mold and remove woody parts. Place in the jar and mix with the salt. Clean down the sides of the jar and add the weight. Alternatively, use a vacuum bag (see p.72).

2. Add an airlock and close the lid securely, making sure it's airtight, or use an elastic band around the clip (see p.67). Alternatively, you will need to burp it daily (see p.67).

3. Leave in a warm place for 2 days. During this time, the salt will leech enough juice from the berries to submerge them. If not, apply more weight.

4. Leave for 1–2 weeks until activity slows, then store in the fridge for up to a month.

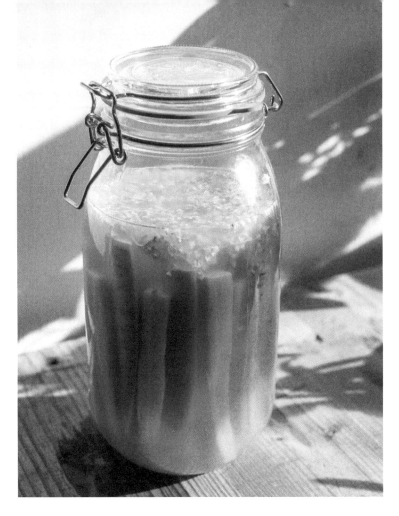

Day 12, fermented carrots
and elderflower.

LACTO CARROTS AND ELDERFLOWER

2-liter jar

glass or ceramic
  weight

airlock or elastic
  band (optional)

or

large vacuum bag

INGREDIENTS

300g baby carrots

70g fresh
  elderflower

4g dried juniper
  berries

26g sea salt (2%)

900g water

This is one of the simplest and most elegant pairings I've come across in fermentation. This springtime recipe is great if you can forage the blossom of elderflower, characterized by its broad crowns of tiny ivory-white flowers. When harvesting elderflowers, make sure to collect them on a cool, sunny morning and use them on the same day, as they wither quickly. Make sure to cut the flowers free from the stem, which contains potentially harmful chemicals, before adding them into this ferment.

1. Clean and top the carrots. Dust the elderflower free of insects. Cut the blossom free from the stems and add them to the jar with the juniper. Place the carrots on top.

2. Dissolve the salt in the water and pour it in. If the ingredients are loose enough to float, put a weight in to hold them down.

3. Add an airlock and close the lid securely, making sure it's airtight, or use an elastic band around the clip (see p.67). Alternatively, you will need to burp it daily (see p.67).

4. Leave the jar somewhere warm, out of direct sunlight for 1 week, then begin trying the ferment to check on the process. The carrots will be ready after 7–14 days, depending on your preference for sourness. Store in the brine for up to 2 months in the fridge.

COOKING
WITH FERMENTS

SIDE DISH
Lacto carrots and elderflower makes a perfect accompaniment to miso soup.

TOPPING
Try serving these lacto carrots on top of whipped feta or hummus.

CHARRED LACTO CARROTS
Char the lacto carrots and drizzle them with an apple balsamic dressing.

LACTO RHUBARB HONEY

EQUIPMENT

1-liter jar

glass or ceramic weight

airlock or elastic band (optional)

or

vacuum bag

INGREDIENTS

220g honey

180g water

12g salt (2%)

170g rhubarb

4g dried juniper berries

4g hibiscus

This recipe makes delicious fermented rhubarb that complements a variety of dishes. However, it is the honey, soured through fermentation and infused with the flavor of rhubarb, that is the star of this recipe. With uses that range from a savory-sweet glaze to ketchups, jams, teas, and poaching liquids, you can apply it to most things. Try adding herbs, spices, or ginger root to broaden the aromatic profile of the honey.

1. Honey itself has too much sugar to ferment, so we have to water it down to make this ferment work. Mix the honey and water together in the sanitized jar with the salt and stir until dissolved.

2. Clean the rhubarb and cut it into ½in (1cm) pieces, then place it in the jar. Add the juniper and hibiscus.

3. Add an airlock and close the lid securely, making sure it's airtight, or use an elastic band around the clip (see p.67). Alternatively, you will need to burp it daily (see p.67).

4. Leave it at room temperature to ferment for 2 weeks, or above 75°F (24°C) for 1 week. Each day, give the jar a little shake to make sure none of the ingredients are left floating above the surface for more than 24 hours.

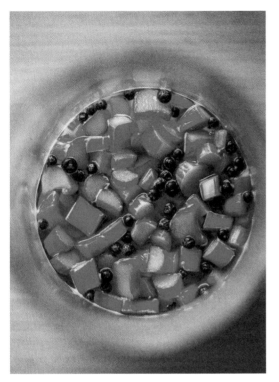

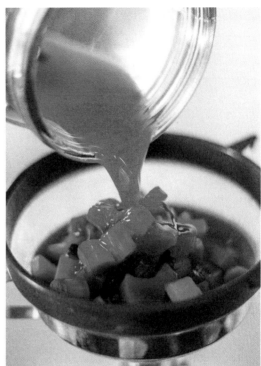

Above Day 1, ingredients floating in honey water brine.

Top right Day 7, filtering the fully fermented rhubarb from the liquid.

Alternatively, if you have a chamber sealer, you can use the vacuum bag method (see p.72), but be warned—clamp sealers won't handle this much liquid, and you'll end up with a sticky mess.

5. After this time, the ferment should be ready to taste. You're looking for something soured, sweet, fruity, and fragrant. The honey will have turned a deep ruby red. Filter the solid ingredients out and use them to make a coulis or add them to a sauce. Bottle the honey and store in a fridge (1 month) or freezer (12 months).

COOKING WITH FERMENTS

DRINKS

Use the honey in small amounts as a tea, as a cordial, or in black coffee.

STEWS AND CASSEROLES

While you might not think it, the sweet fruitiness of the honey ferment complements sauces and stews—the more savory, the better.

BREAKFAST

Mix some of the leftover rhubarb into a compote to use as a topping for yogurt, cereal, or pancakes.

SAUCES

A small amount of honey will transform sweet, creamy sauces and custards.

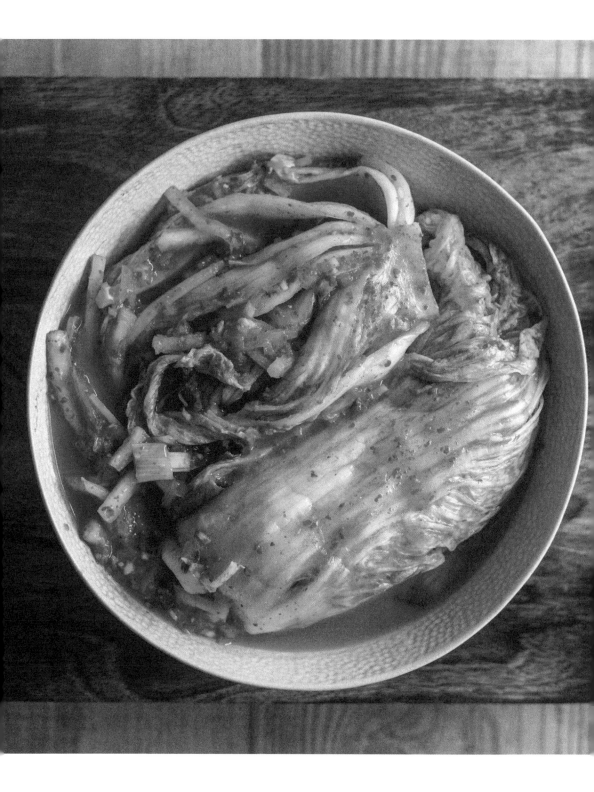

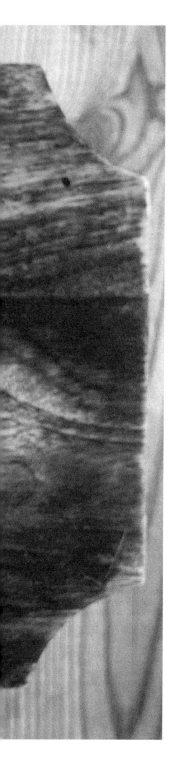

Rustic, fully fermented
Baechu kimchi in a bowl.

KIMCHI

Kimchi has become a global superstar in recent years, and deservedly so. But like most fermentation techniques, it comes from humble origins, with many beautiful regional variations. What began as a means to store crops over winter has become a form of culinary and cultural expression. With help from my friend Kim Jihyun, known as Kimmy, the owner of Kimchi&Radish, here are some of my favorites.

Kimchi has
become a form
of culinary
and cultural
expression.

NABAK KIMCHI

This is a type of water kimchi, made with thin slices of vegetables, and it most closely resembles the kind of lacto fermentation featured in this book. This short-lived kimchi's full name is *nabak sseolgi* (나박썰기), which refers to the way the ingredients are cut. Prized for being refreshing, it's often served ice cold with noodles during the summer. The salt is 2 percent of the combined ingredients, including the water.

EQUIPMENT

3-liter jar or crock

INGREDIENTS

650g radish
(preferably
daikon/mooli,
or any large,
mild-tasting
variety)

1 carrot (120g)

500g cabbage
(preferably napa)

80g salt (2%)

1 tbsp gochugaru
(optional)

120g warm water
(optional)

1 apple or pear
(170g)

3 garlic cloves
(20g)

3 spring onions
(15g)

20g ginger root

1 bunch of minari
(see Fermenter's
Note)

about 2.3kg water

1. Clean the radish and carrot—no need to peel them. Cut the radish into thin pieces, roughly ¾–1¼in (2 × 3cm) and only a few millimeters thick. Remove the cabbage leaves from the stem and give them a quick wash. Cut the cabbage leaves into 1¼in (3cm) pieces.

2. Put the cabbage in a bowl with the radish and salt. Toss the ingredients around, then cover and leave somewhere at room temperature for 30 minutes to draw the water out.

3. While you wait, if you're being traditional, cut three little V-shaped grooves along the length of the carrot, then chop it up into ⅛in (3mm) disks to make them look like flower petals. Add the carrot to the bowl with the cabbage and radish.

4. Soak the gochugaru in the warm water to make a spicy shot. Leave to infuse for 20 minutes. If you don't like spice, you can skip this step.

5. Peel and core the apple or pear and cut into small pieces. Thinly slice the remaining ingredients and put them all into the bowl with the cabbage and mix well.

6. Pack them all into the jar or crock, along with the water released from them and any undissolved salt.

7. Top up the container with enough of the fresh, cold water to cover everything, leaving enough room for the shot of gochugaru, if using.

8. Filter out the gochugaru, if used, and add the golden red liquid to the jar. Close the lid and leave to ferment for just 2–3 days before storing in a fridge for up to 2 weeks.

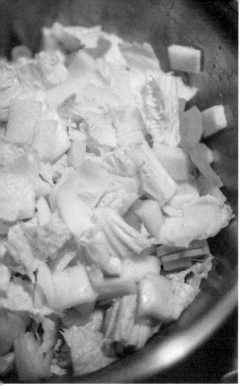

Above What makes Nabak special is the way each ingredient is cut, epitomized by the shape of the carrot slices.

Right Day 3, prior to refrigeration.

BRINED POTATO WEDGES

Cut a few baking potatoes into wedges, pack them into a container, and cover with the leftover brine. Place them in a fridge overnight before patting them dry and baking them the next day as you would regular oven-baked wedges.

●

FERMENTER'S NOTE

If you struggle to source minari (also called water dropwort, water celery, or Chinese celery) and aren't an experienced forager, I'd recommend using fresh flat-leaf parsley instead.

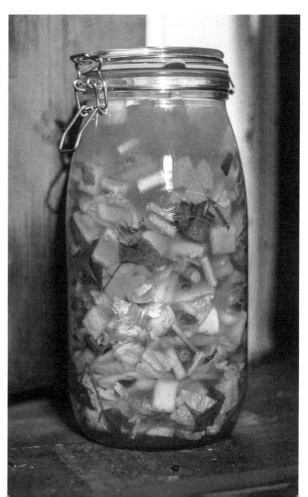

BAECHU
KIMCHI

EQUIPMENT

1-liter lunch box

INGREDIENTS

4–5 napa cabbages
or other cabbages
(3kg)

150g salt

50g glutinous rice
flour

450g water

30g sugar or honey

1 medium brown
onion

20g ginger root

50g fermented
salted shrimp or
30g sweet white
miso

80g fish sauce or
vegan fish sauce

80g gochugaru
(optional)

440g daikon/mooli

1 carrot (120g)

100g spring onions

1 bunch of minari
(see Fermenter's
Note, p.91)

Yes, this is THAT kimchi you're all familiar with. Baechu
(배추김치), also called napa cabbage, is the key ingredient
in this quintessential kimchi you've seen lining the shelves at
the store, but homemade is infinitely better. In Korea, there is
a term "*son-mat*" (손맛), literally meaning "hand taste," which
refers to the superior taste of something made by hand and
the love that labor imparts. This phrase was published in
the front of Sandro Katz's world-famous book, *The Art of
Fermentation*, but I feel it is especially relevant to kimchi.

If you aren't a fan of spice, make this recipe without the
gochugaru to make "white kimchi" or *baek kimchi* (백김치).

Note that salt is handled a little differently in this recipe.
To begin with, salt is used to draw moisture from the
cabbage, then it is washed off. Some salt remains, and
the rest is made up with salty ingredients (fish sauce and
salted shrimp or miso). For this reason, I've left out the
guidance percentage. Instead, I'd advise you to scale the
quantities of the recipe to suit your needs.

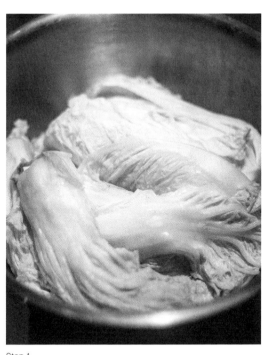

Step 1.

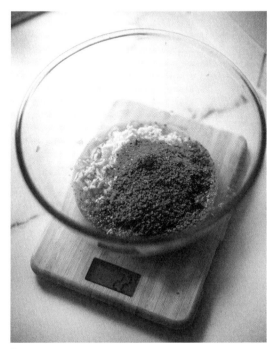

Step 4.

● FERMENTER'S NOTE

For a plant-based version, swap the fish sauce for a vegan fish sauce or light soy sauce, and use miso instead of shrimp. If you can't find a vegan fish sauce, you can use white soy sauce and seaweed instead.

1. To begin, cut the woody stem of the cabbages off flush to the lowest leaves, but keep the core intact to hold the cabbage together. Cut a cross through the stem of each cabbage and tear them into quarters by hand, down the length. Salt liberally between each layer of leaf and pile them into a large mixing bowl. Cover and leave for 30 minutes–1 hour.

2. While you wait, mix the glutinous rice flour with 100g water to make a thick paste, then add the remaining 350g water and cook over medium-high heat for 10 minutes, stirring continuously to stop the mixture from clumping at the base of the pan, until the paste is thick and bubbling.

3. Add the sugar or honey, stir to dissolve, then remove the pan from the heat. Leave to cool completely.

4. Mince the onion, ginger, and fermented salted shrimp into a paste and add it into a second bowl with the fish sauce and gochugaru, if using.

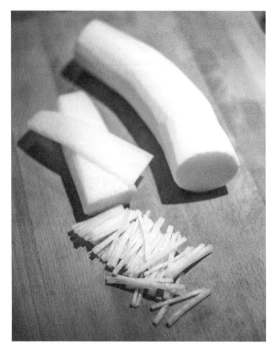

Step 5, julienned daikon.

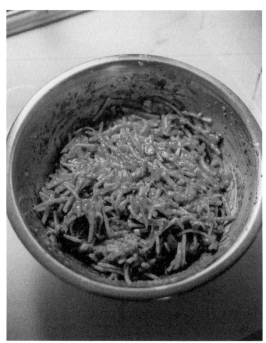

Step 5, mixed vegetables and kimchi paste.

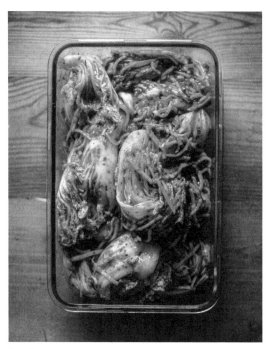

Step 7.

5. Julienne the daikon and carrot into matchsticks and slice the spring onions and minari into ½in (1cm) pieces. Add to the bowl of kimchi paste, along with the cooled rice paste. Mix together and set aside.

6. Remove the remaining stem from the softened cabbage, but leave enough intact to hold the layers of cabbage together. Rinse the salt off, then rub each layer with a handful of kimchi paste from the other bowl. Repeat this until every layer of every piece of cabbage is red with gochugaru or well covered.

7. Roll them up and pack them tightly into a lunch box. Pour any remaining kimchi paste over the top and rub it in, then secure the lid onto the lunch box.

8. Leave it at room temperature (68–77°F/ 20–25°C) for 1–2 days. Fermentation will kick in and bulge the lid, so make sure to release the pressure by opening it once a day.

9. Once the mixture looks more liquidy and bubbles when pressed, transfer the whole box to the fridge and let it age. It is ready to eat after 2–3 days in the fridge, but will mature gradually for a month. Keep in the fridge and use within 2 months.

COOKING WITH FERMENTS

DEHYDRATED KIMCHI POWDER

Dehydrate leftover kimchi for 12 hours at 113°F (45°C), then crush or blend it into a coarse powder and store at room temperature in an airtight container. Use it like a regular spice powder, or mix with salt to make a flavored salt to finish off recipes with a kimchi kick.

BRAISED KIMCHI

Charring and braising kimchi changes its flavor completely into something rich, umami, and delicious.

KIMCHI AND TAHINI UDON

Cook udon noodles according to the package instructions and, when the noodles are almost done, add some kimchi to a hot frying pan with a little sunflower oil, tahini, some yeast flakes, and a little water to loosen the mixture up. Stir in the noodles and serve with nori and sprouted beans.

KIMCHI BROTH

Add kimchi to broths and soups after removing them from the heat to retain crunch and sourness, and finish with toasted sesame seeds.

KIMCHI GRILLED CHEESE

I couldn't miss this one. If you're one of the few people who haven't tried it yet, place some kimchi in a grilled cheese and cook until the cheese is melted. It's very naughty and absolutely delicious.

SIDE DISH

Treat as a tasty bowl of pickled vegetables as a side to meals.

KIMCHI RICE SALAD

Finely chop fully aged kimchi and mix it into cold, cooked rice. Top with sesame and nigella seeds for a delicious salad.

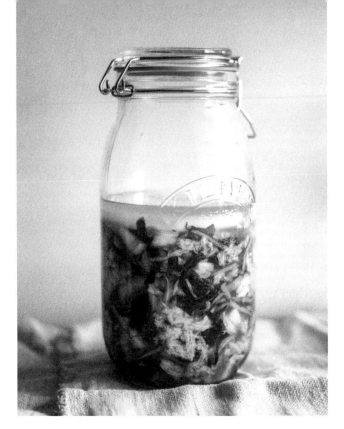

Day 1 (left) and day 15 (right).

SAUERKRAUT

EQUIPMENT

4-liter jar or crock

glass or ceramic
  weight

airlock or elastic
  band (optional)

INGREDIENTS

2–3 large cabbages
  (2.5kg)

55g sea salt (2%)

10g dried juniper
  berries

This is one of the most famous lacto ferments in Europe, and one I have fond memories of making in bulk at a restaurant I worked in. Hundreds of hours of my life have been spent massaging salt into shredded cabbage. Then we'd leave it all in a quiet corner in the cellar for months until the whole room smelled of delicious tangy cabbage.

This recipe is a scaled-down version of what we used to make, with some dried juniper berries to add a fun spin. The process of making sauerkraut is also a wonderful way to use waste produce, such as broccoli and kale stems, so once you've got the basics, experiment and make your own glorious discoveries.

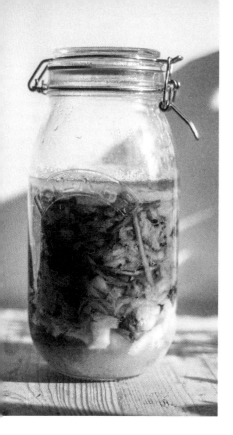

●
FERMENTER'S NOTE
Try adding other ingredients to the cabbage: beets, ginger, and lemon all make great additions and fun colors.

1. Begin by cutting the cabbages into manageable pieces and removing any hard, woody stems. Rinse these pieces under cold water and shred them using a knife or mandoline. Depending on your preference for crunch, you can leave them thick or slice very thinly.

2. Once shredded, put the cabbage into a large mixing bowl and add the salt. With both hands, massage the salt into the cabbage, bruising the leaves. This will take 5–10 minutes and might make your hands cramp. You'll notice that the cabbage releases a lot of water. This will dissolve the salt and become the fermenting brine, so make sure not to spill any.

3. Once the cabbage is suitably floppy, cram it into the jar as tightly as you can and pour all the salty water in, too. Apply a fermentation weight to the top, ideally enough to bring the liquid level above the cabbage, although this will continue to rise over the next day as the salt draws more water from the leaves. If you struggle to keep the small pieces of cabbage under the weight, lay a sheet of parchment paper over the surface, then place the weight on top.

4. Add an airlock and close the lid securely, making sure it's airtight, or use an elastic band around the clip (see p.67). Alternatively, you will need to burp it daily (see p.67).

5. Leave somewhere at room temperature, out of direct sunlight, for 1 month. If using a completely sealed container, remember to open the lid daily to release the build-up of carbon dioxide.

6. Once the cabbage has fermented for a month, it will be deliciously tangy and sour. At this stage, move it to a fridge or cool cellar, where it will keep for 6–7 months.

EQUIPMENT

2.5-liter jar

airlock or elastic
band (optional)

2 × 750ml bottles

INGREDIENTS

700g young green
pine cones

1.4kg raw brown
sugar (double the
weight of pine
cones)

Try this for the ultimate flavor of the forest and an opportunity to get out of the kitchen and forage. Pine cones, specifically from the Scots pine (*Pinus sylvestris*), are an old and largely forgotten food in the UK, but to me, they symbolize a connection to the Caledonian forest. Scots pine can be identified by the two pink balls that appear on the end of the stem during spring and early summer. However, you can use any edible varieties.

Once made, you can store the syrup at room temperature, as it is shelf stable, but the best flavor will be preserved if kept in a fridge.

1. Inspect the pine cones for damage or signs of pests, and gently wash them if required.

2. Put them in a large bowl with twice their weight in sugar (this can be any kind of brown sugar, but I find raw has the best flavor), give them a mix, then pack them into the jar.

3. Add an airlock and close the lid securely, making sure it's airtight, or use an elastic band around the clip (see p.67). Alternatively, you will need to burp it daily (see p.67).

PINE CONE SYRUP

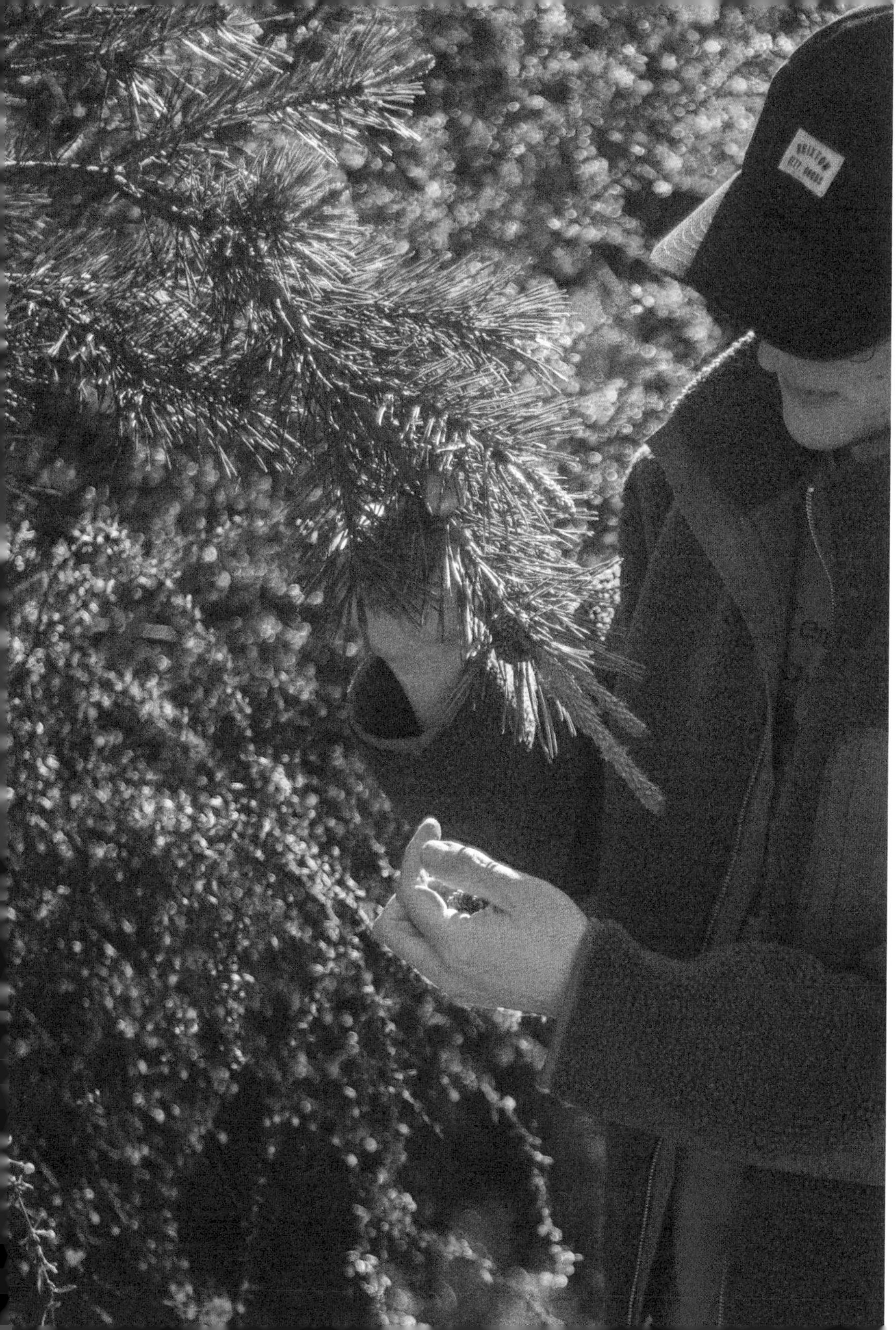

4. Put on a sunny windowsill. The sun helps prevent mold, but you should also give the jar a daily shake for the first 2 weeks once the sap has dissolved the sugar into a liquid.

5. Once the sugar dissolves, you will have more room in the jar. Feel free to top it up with more pine cones and sugar to make the most of the space, but you don't have to.

6. After the activity slows right down (it will be bubbling less), after 1–2 months, pour it all into a saucepan, scraping out any undissolved sugar, and bring all of it to a rapid simmer for 2 minutes. Stir to dissolve the remaining sugar, then strain out the cones (see opposite for using the cones).

7. Bottle the syrup while piping hot. Secure the lids, then leave to cool at room temperature. Store for up to 1 year at room temperature and keep in a fridge once opened.

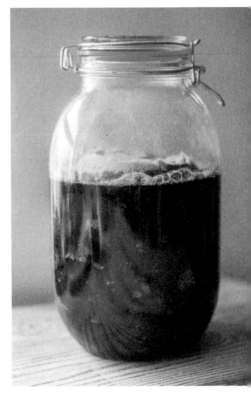

Step 5, the sugar slowly dissolving in the sap.

COOKING WITH FERMENTS

PANCAKE TOPPING

My favorite way to enjoy pine cone syrup is drizzled over pancakes.

PAIR WITH SOFT CHEESES

Drizzle pine cone syrup over soft cheeses, such as brie, ricotta, and young goat cheese.

SALAD DRESSINGS

Mix the syrup with oil and vinegar to make incredible dressings.

HONEY ALTERNATIVE

Use the syrup instead of floral honey.

STICKY GLAZE

Use the syrup as a glaze for meats and mushrooms by loosening with a splash of vinegar, whisky, or melted butter.

SWEET CREAM

Whip pine cone syrup into cream to serve with desserts, tarts, and fruit salads.

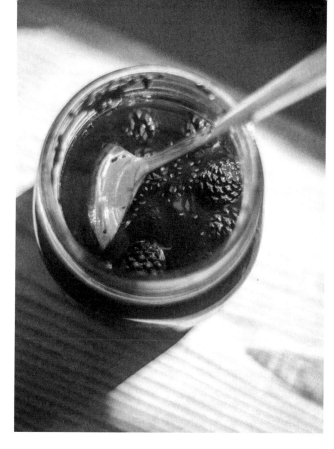

Candied pine cones
in resin and sugar.

CANDIED PINE CONES

Don't throw away your leftover pine cones; candy them in sugar for a soft-toffee-textured pine treat.

EQUIPMENT

cartouche
(parchment paper
lid)

INGREDIENTS

570g leftover
pine cones
(see pp.98–100)

625g white sugar

1.4kg water

1. Put the leftover pine cones back in the saucepan with the white sugar and water. They will be lighter now they've lost sap to the syrup, but there is still flavor in resin that can be extracted. Bring the pan to a rapid boil, then reduce to a simmer and place the cartouche over the surface.

2. Simmer for 3 hours, then check if it's ready by spooning a small amount of the liquid onto a cold plate. If it doesn't thicken to the consistency of syrup, then continue to cook for another 20–30 minutes uncovered and try again.

3. Once it is thick, transfer the cones and the liquid to an airtight jar in the fridge, adding them while hot. Store for up to 3 months. Enjoy them like candy.

BLACK GARLIC

EQUIPMENT

vacuum bag,
  aluminum foil,
  or beeswax

multicooker or rice
  cooker

INGREDIENTS

6 bulbs garlic

An absolute legend in the culinary world, black garlic is deeply umami with distinct notes of tamarind and liquorice. In fermentation, we are most concerned with time and temperature to control the alteration of ingredients via microbial activity. But in black garlic, we stray into the world of aging. By holding it at 140°F (60°C) for 6–8 weeks, we cause a chemical reaction between the sugars and amino acids, altering the composition, flavor, and color of the ingredient. While some might argue that this process isn't fermentation and doesn't deserve a place in this book, I believe the process is worth including due to the extraordinary flavor and nutrition it yields and overlap in specialty equipment.

Step 1, fresh garlic
in a vacuum bag.

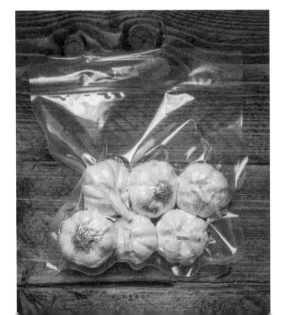

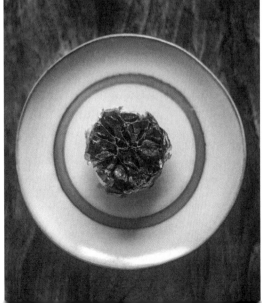

1. The key to this process is warmth and moisture. By using a vacuum sealer or tightly wrapped aluminum foil, or dipping in melted beeswax, we can trap the moisture of the garlic within as we hold it at 140°F (60°C) for the duration of the aging process. To do this, most multicookers or rice cookers come with a "keep warm" setting. It's important to check your exact model doesn't stray above or below this temperature, as this will leave the garlic vulnerable to spoilage or burning. The melting point of beeswax is 144°F (62°C), so it's even more important to not stray too high if you're using this approach.

2. Once the garlic is securely sealed, place a small plate or upturned bowl in the bottom of the cooker to form a barrier and stop the garlic burning, then place it on top and set to "keep warm." Place it somewhere out of the way and set a reminder to check it after 6–8 weeks.

3. The black garlic is done when the cloves are black and soft like dates, with a rich balsamic note. At this stage, it can be stored in an airtight container for 3 months in a cabinet or 6 months in a fridge.

●
FERMENTER'S NOTE

This exact same process can be applied to many fruits, vegetables, and nuts to unlock transformative flavors. When using this technique for fruits, peel first and take care not to overhandle. The fruit becomes very soft after the first week.

COOKING WITH FERMENTS

SAUCES
Cook into sauces by hydrating a few cloves in warm water and blending them into any sauce of your choice— I especially love black garlic BBQ sauce or mole.

DIPS
Blend into black turtle bean hummus with plenty of lemon and salt, or mince and add into salsas.

SALAD DRESSINGS
Combine with one part balsamic vinegar and two parts olive oil and blend to make a dressing.

STEWS
Transform creamy, tomato, and beef stews with a few cloves sliced and slowly cooked.

BLACK GARLIC MAYONNAISE
Blend into mayonnaise for one of the fanciest aioli you'll ever eat.

BLACK GARLIC ICE CREAM
Hear me out …. Mix just a small amount into vanilla, honey, or chocolate ice cream, offering a rich umami flavor you never knew was lacking from regular ice cream.

LACTIC ACID BACTE*RIA* AND DAIRY

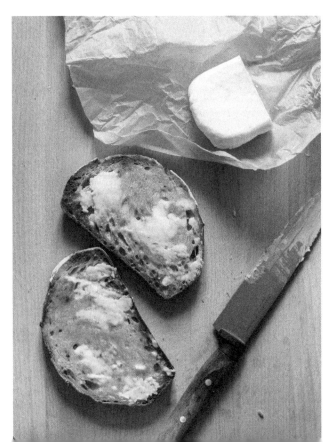

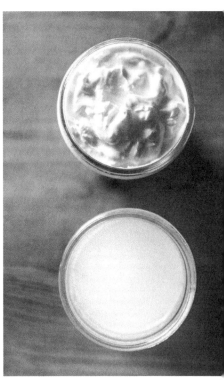

Left Cultured butter.

Above Yogurt and whey.

Lactic acid bacteria is also responsible for some of our most celebrated dairy foods. *Lactobacillus bulgaricus* and *Streptococcus thermophilus* (this is not the same variety as *Streptococcus pyogenes*, which is a bacterial pathogen) both create yogurt and are responsible for the classic sour tanginess, as well as thickening the milk. Most of the recipes within each chapter are arranged based on the length of time it takes to make them, but I've kept this small handful of dairy- and whey-based ferments in a grouping of their own. Both whey and buttermilk are leftover products of these processes, and whey can be included in all of the previous lacto ferment recipes in place of 20 percent of the added water. Buttermilk can be used in baking, pancakes, or batters or as a delicious marinade for mushroom and animal proteins thanks to its acidity.

HOMEMADE
YOGURT

EQUIPMENT

thermometer

thick blanket, insulated box, or hot-water bottle

small jar (to store yogurt in for next time)

straining bag or large dish towel

INGREDIENTS

2 liters whole milk (non-homogenized)

2 tbsp natural yogurt

Nothing beats fresh, homemade yogurt. For a start, it's only two ingredients. And you can avoid the stabilizers, thickeners, and preservatives found in a lot of store-bought options. While cheese-making is a whole book in its own right, yogurt is a quick and easy ferment that can be enjoyed as part of other recipes, both sweet and savory. The presence of milk also aids the beneficial bacteria in their passage through your stomach on their way to their new home in your intestine.

If you have a yogurt machine or multicooker with a fermentation setting, then you'll be able to fine-tune the results for this recipe. If not, I suggest using whatever you have on hand (an insulated box, a thick blanket, or even a hot-water bottle).

The rise in popularity of plant-based milk alternatives may leave some wondering if it's possible to turn them into yogurt using the same recipe. While I have yet to find results that truly satisfy me, you can indeed do it. I've found the texture to be a little off, but the best results are from homemade plant milks, such as cashew, hazelnut, or soy.

1. Bring the milk to a boil over medium heat, stirring constantly. When the milk reaches boiling point, remove it from the heat. Pour it into a bowl and leave it to cool for 30 minutes until it's 104–113°F (40–45°C).

2. Allow the natural yogurt from the fridge to warm to room temperature during this time.

3. Once the milk has cooled, pour 200ml into the yogurt and stir them together to loosen the yogurt, then add the mixture back into the bowl and stir.

4. You now have two options: cover with a loose-fitting lid (such as a plate) that allows oxygen in, and you'll have a more complex, slightly cheesy yogurt; or cover with an airtight lid, which will force anaerobic fermentation to focus purely on making lactic acid. The aerobic one tends to be a more traditional flavor, while anaerobic is what you'll commonly find in stores. I tend to go aerobic, but the cheesiness doesn't suit every application. Put the bowl somewhere warm, wrapped in a thick blanket, or in an insulated box or in the oven (turned off) with a hot-water bottle. Leave overnight for 9 hours.

5. Move it into the fridge the following day for another 20–24 hours.

6. Congratulations, you now have yogurt. Place about 100g of this runny natural yogurt into an airtight container and store it in the fridge for next time. It will keep for 1 week.

7. With the rest, you can either enjoy it as is or strain it and remove some of the whey (the yellowish liquid) in order to thicken it. Personally, I prefer thick yogurt. I also love using whey in other lacto ferments. So it's a win-win. To strain the yogurt, hang it in a secure, sanitized cloth above a clean bowl. This can be done in a fridge or at room temperature. It will take about a day to get to a super-thick, creamy consistency. Store it back in the fridge again afterward; strained yogurt will last for 2–3 weeks in the fridge.

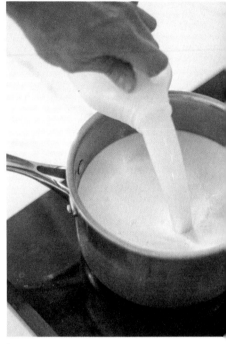

Step 1.

COOKING WITH FERMENTS

YOGURT AND CUCUMBER

Mixed the yogurt with sliced cucumber, walnuts, raisins, sliced spring onions, mint, dill, and salt and top with fresh or dried rose petals, mixed peppercorns, and a drizzle of extra virgin olive oil.

WHEY LOAF

Replace the water in bread dough with yogurt whey for a delicious whey loaf.

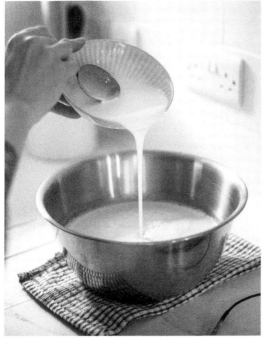

Step 3.

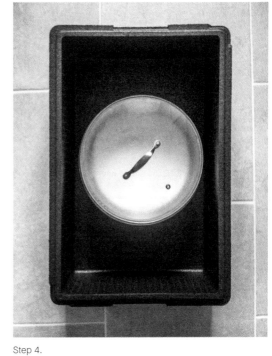

Step 4.

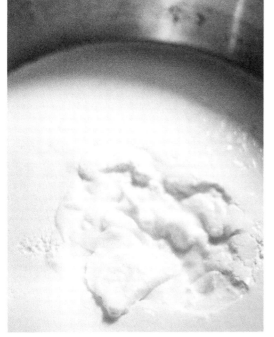

Step 6.

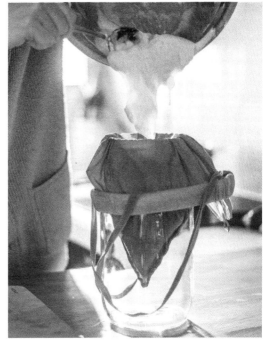

Step 7.

CULTURED BUTTER

I cannot emphasize enough—if you're a fan of butter, you have to try this recipe. It's insanely easy, too. I first learned how to make butter back when I was a kid at Acton Scott farm in Shropshire. It's one of those "ye olde" practices that's easy to fall in love with, but fermenting the cream before turning it into butter is a game-changer.

EQUIPMENT

butter churner
(optional)

INGREDIENTS

800ml heavy cream

100g homemade
yogurt (see
pp.105–107 or use
natural yogurt)

10g salt

1. Pour the heavy cream into a large, clean bowl. Add the yogurt and mix until there are no lumps.

2. Cover with a cloth and leave to ferment at room temperature for 24 hours. Signs of activity are bubbles appearing on the surface; a tangy, cheesy smell; and the cream will set. (Congratulations, you've now learned how to make crème fraîche.)

3. Once fermented, spoon the mixture into a butter churner (or use a stand mixer or mixing bowl and hand-held electric whisk) and churn on high speed for 10 minutes. Keep an eye on it and reduce the speed in the last few minutes as the butter forms, releasing the buttermilk, a watery liquid that will go everywhere if the mixer is left on high speed. When this happens, hook the butter from the buttermilk and give it a squeeze to release excess liquid.

4. Wash it in ice-cold water by gently folding and squeezing it between your hands to remove as much buttermilk as possible; this will help extend its shelf life.

5. Salt and form the butter, then wrap it in parchment paper and store it in the fridge. If done correctly, it should last 3 weeks (or freeze for 9 months).

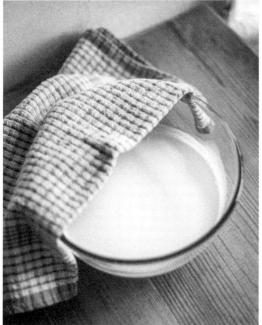

Step 1.

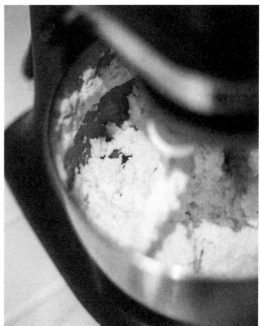

Step 3.

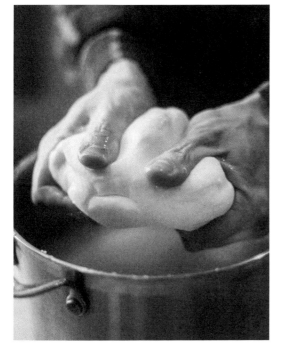

Step 4.

COOKING WITH FERMENTS

BUTTER SUBSTITUTION

You can use cultured butter on toast, in garlic bread, for your sandwiches and grilled cheese, in roux, in pastry, and even in cakes. You can use it for frying shrimp and grilling oysters or for making confit garlic. Basically, anything you normally love making with a healthy knob of butter!

COMPOUND BUTTER

The world of compound butter is vast, but at its core, it simply means butter mixed with something else, such as herbs, spices, seaweed, wild garlic, citrus peel, flower and blossom petals, yeast extract, shio kōji, and (of course) miso.

Day 1 (left) and day 14 (right), the colors yellow and the liquid clouds before turning clear again.

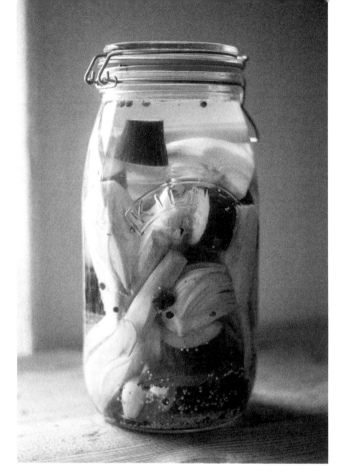

WHEY
PICK*LES*

So what to do with all that delicious whey from yogurt-making? Filled to the brim with lively beneficial microbes, whey is the perfect ingredient to kick-start all your lacto ferments. In fact, you can substitute some of the water (roughly 5–10 percent) for whey in lacto ferments and they will spring into action. Whey will impart a slight cheesy tang to ingredients, which really suits things like cauliflower and cabbage. I haven't given weights here, but instead have provided instructions for you to calculate the salt based on the weight of the ingredients you use.

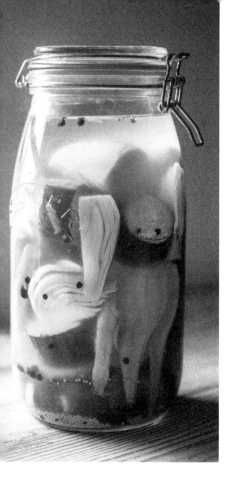

1. Clean and prepare the ingredients. Remove ¾in (2cm) of the flowering head of the cucumbers (which is the end without a bit of stem sticking out) and cut the cucumbers into 1¼in (3cm) chunks. Remove the hard stem of the fennel and cut them into 5–6 wedges. I find a ferment like this is easier to weigh down when not cut too finely. Peel the garlic.

2. Tare the scales to the weight of the jar. Add all the ingredients except the salt, then add enough water to cover. Take note of the weight. Multiply this number by 0.02 to calculate the amount of salt to add, pour it in, close the lid, and shake until it's dissolved. Open the lid again and add a weight to keep the ingredients submerged.

3. Leave the jar somewhere at 68–86°F (20–30°C) for 2 weeks, opening the jar daily to release the build-up of carbon dioxide. Start tasting after a week to check on the progress and move it to a fridge once it's your desired level of sourness. Once made, the ingredients make a great addition to sandwiches, grilled cheese, burgers, BBQ (charred or fresh off the grill), and salads.

EQUIPMENT

3-liter clip-top jar

food-safe bag or weight

INGREDIENTS

3 fennel bulbs

2 cucumbers

5 garlic cloves

1 tbsp yellow mustard seeds

1 tbsp peppercorns

1 bay leaf

200g yogurt whey (see p.106)

salt (2%)

●
FERMENTER'S NOTE

Sometimes garlic can turn blue or green when exposed to an acidic environment. This is perfectly normal and has no negative effects on flavor or health. This happens due to the breakdown of cells, giving enzymes access to the sulfur in garlic, a process that results in microscopic ring structures that absorb light differently, giving the garlic its blue or green hue.

FERMENTED GRAINS *IN* WHEY

My good friend, chef Nathan Davies, showed me this incredible recipe for fermenting local grain in water, salt, and whey. When done properly, this technique creates chewy, springy, delicious grains that can be cooked into broths and breads, or served as Nathan does, cooked in miso butter (see compound butter, p.109).

EQUIPMENT

2-liter jar

glass weight
  (optional)

airlock

INGREDIENTS

500g spelt, wheat,
  and/or barley

500g water

500g yogurt whey
  (see p.106)

30g sea salt (2%)

1. Tare the scales to the weight of the jar. Fill the jar with either a single type of grain or a mixture and top up with half water and half yogurt whey.

2. Measure and add the salt, then mix until the salt is dissolved. If necessary, weigh the grains down with a glass weight (or fill a vacuum bag with water and add to the top).

3. Secure with an airlock and leave at 68°F (20°C) for a month until the pH reaches 3.5.

4. Move it to the fridge, either in the same jar, or, to save fridge space, vacuum seal it with the fermentation brine. It can be used right away or aged in the fridge for up to 6 months.

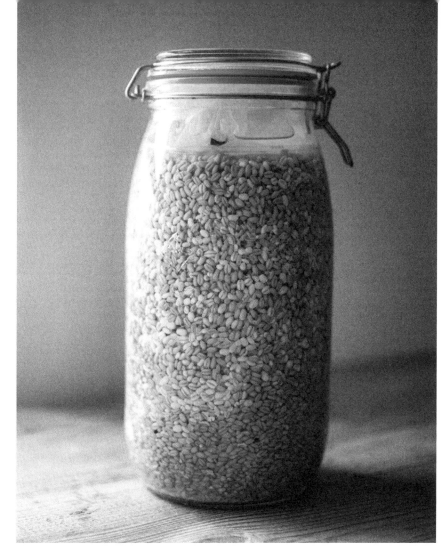

Fermented grains ready to pack and age in the fridge.

●
FERMENTER'S NOTE

When starting a fresh batch, inoculate with some of the liquid from a previous batch. This will kick the ferment into gear quickly and produce extra-springy, chewy grain.

COOKING WITH FERMENTS

BREAD

Add a handful of fermented grains into bread dough after the first proof and bake as usual.

BROTHS

Cook into broths and stews for a chewy, springy texture and savory, acidic pop.

Yeasts occupy the mid scale in our microscopic journey. They are larger than bacteria but smaller and less complex than mold. Within food, yeasts are most commonly responsible for the production of alcohols such as beer, cider, wine, and mead, as well as breads and some pastries. But they are also present in drinks such as kombucha, where they form part of a symbiotic relationship with bacteria, which makes such ferments possible.

YEAST

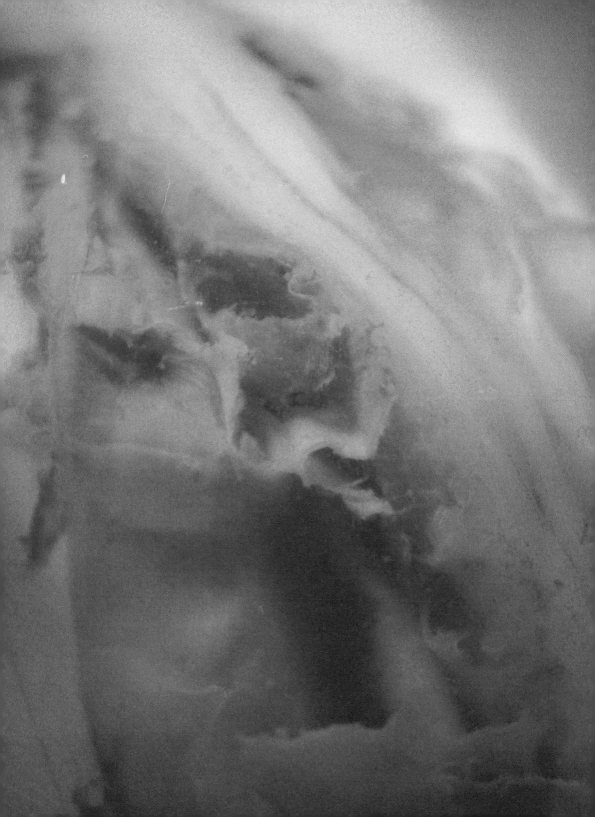

SUGAR AND YEAST

Food for all the yeasts in the following recipes is sugar dissolved in liquid, which explains why *Saccharomyces*, a genus of fungi including many species of yeast, means "sugar fungus" in Greek. *Saccharomyces* is responsible for baker's yeast, sourdough starters, and the brewing of alcoholic beverages. It encompasses a broad range of microbes and flavors, including wild yeasts such as *Saccharomyces paradoxus* and *Saccharomyces bayanus*, which are both used in winemaking, as well as varieties that are used in probiotic medicine.

For this book, I'll focus more on the production of alcohol and leave bread out of it (see p218 for my bread book recommendations). I'll list the alcohol level (ABV) for guidance. This is a rough estimate and can vary depending on the temperature and conditions of your fermentation.

SACCHAROMYCES

These single-celled fungal organisms called yeast feed on sugar dissolved in liquid, producing ethanol and carbon dioxide.

As we cannot completely rule out smaller players, this is lactic acid bacteria (LAB), shown as many times smaller in comparison to yeast.

Yeast cells have a vacuole that makes up roughly 25 percent of their total size and helps regulate pH and ion homeostasis.

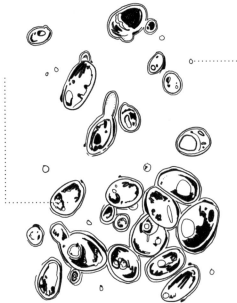

SMALLER PLAYERS

As we increase in size of microorganisms, it becomes difficult to rule out the involvement of smaller players. For a lot of the recipes in this chapter, it's worth mentioning that many of the lactic acid bacteria (LAB) from the previous chapter also contribute.

MEASURING SUGAR

It is very important we have a means to measure the sugar quantity in the liquid accurately so we know how much the yeast has to feed on, and, more importantly, monitor the production of alcohol and acid (both of which make these ferments safe).

REFRACTOMETERS

The most simple way to do this is with a refractometer (see p.51), which is both affordable and easy to use. Dissolved sugars alter the optical properties of water by changing the angle that light passes through it. Using a refractometer, we are able to observe the extent of this change and translate it to a number (degrees Brix), giving us a good idea of how much sugar is dissolved within the liquid.

MEASURING DEGREES BRIX (°BX) USING A REFRACTOMETER

A degree brix is the measure of the angle of light passing through water, expressed as a numerical value.

One degree Brix (1°Bx) corresponds to 1g sucrose in 100g water, representing a percentage by mass. Therefore, 1 part sucrose to 1 part water has a measurement of 50°Bx. Brix itself isn't a measurement, but a scale that correlates to the specific gravity of the solution. The density of sugar syrup and regular water differ. The more sugar, the higher the specific gravity, which happens to also change the angle of light passing through it. Using a refractometer, we can observe the angle and translate this to a numerical value indicating the sweetness of a liquid. If this sounds overly complex, fear not. It simply involves placing a drop of liquid on one end of a small telescope-looking object, then looking through it to see which number it reads.

This is useful if I need to calculate how much sugar to add to berry juice when making wine or how much sugar is left in a fermented kombucha, for example.

However, other dissolvable solids, such as salt, can also affect the reading, which will raise the degrees of refraction faster than sugar. So it's important to measure while a solution contains only sugar, if you require the addition of other ingredients.

HYDROMETERS

The increased density of water containing dissolved sugar also makes it possible to use another measuring device, a hydrometer (see p.50). This is very useful, affordable, and simple to use. A hydrometer is lowered into water, displacing a degree of water. Where the liquid surface reaches on the hydrometer tells us how dense the liquid is: the higher the density reading, the higher the sugar content (and lower alcohol content); the lower the density reading, the lower the sugar content (and the higher the alcohol levels).

MEASURING ABV USING A HYDROMETER

When a batch of fresh alcohol is made, prior to fermentation, drop the hydrometer in when the liquid is at 68°F (20°C) and take note of the exact number at the surface of the liquid. There is usually guidance printed on the hydrometer itself to help with starting and end points. Ferment the liquid until activity slows, then take another reading. Notice how much

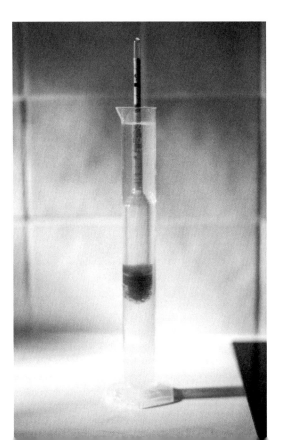
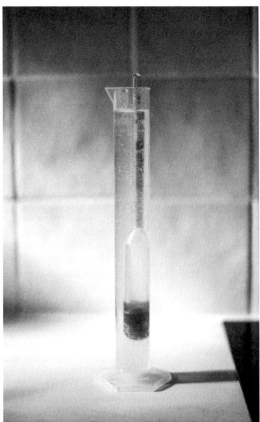

Too much sugar, and yeast will go wild.

lower the hydrometer drops now the sugar has been converted. Subtract the final reading from the original one you made note of, then multiply by 131.25 to calculate the ABV. For example, if a wine starts with a reading of 1.075 and ends at 0.985, the difference is 0.09. Multiply this by 131.25 and the ABV is 11.8 percent.

Most hydrometers come with all the relevant safety information and guidance on correct usage; however, they don't always say to make sure the alcohol being tested is 68°F (20°C) and uncarbonated. If you've made a sparkling beverage, pour some out and let it go flat before taking measurements, as the bubbles can skew results.

While it is possible to follow all the recipes in this book without a refractometer, I'd recommend you get a hydrometer. If you're interested in developing your own recipes, it will be a valuable asset.

OPTIMUM SWEETNESS
There can be too much of a good thing. Too much sugar, and yeast will go wild, producing overly acidic or alcoholic concoctions, and knock itself into dormancy. Far too much, and nothing will happen at all (which is why honey is shelf stable, averaging a sugar content of 82 percent). Too little sugar, and yeast will run out of food and starve. For the recipes in this chapter, I've specified what works as a sweet spot for ferments in my climate and my preference of outcome. The following recipes will work wherever you live, but I encourage you to experiment and fine-tune the results to your own taste.

It's also important to know that not all sweetness comes from sugar, and yeast won't be able to feed off alternative sweeteners.

On the left, the hydrometer shows a high buoyancy, indicating high amounts of dissolved sugar. On the right, the hydrometer drops much lower postfermentation. This is thanks to the yeast converting the sugar to ethanol, lowering the liquid's buoyancy.

WILD YEAST

One of the most wonderful discoveries I've made is the never-ending flavors of wild yeast cultures. Similar to the lactic acid fermentation in the previous chapter, which makes use of the bacteria naturally living on the ingredients and ourselves, wild yeasts are also everywhere and waiting for the ideal conditions to thrive. My first steps into the world of alcohol were armed with a small sachet of brewer's yeast, which is manufactured to produce a specific result every time. Wild yeast, by contrast, is almost impossible to recreate from batch to batch. The beauty in this is a world of flavor that offers a direct and true sensory experience of the microbiology living locally to us and our produce.

The downside is that not all results are delicious from the moment you first sip them. Instead, they require an additional step: mixology. Through the delicate art of combining flavors, you can balance overly harsh flavors and elevate subtle but beautiful undertones. This can be done with additional ingredients by mixing multiple batches of alcohol on the go that pair with one another harmoniously, or even something as simple as serving the drink chilled, which also alters how we perceive its flavor. As you make your way through this chapter, you'll move through wild yeast recipes to recipes that are inoculated with specific cultures of selected yeast, ranging from kombucha SCOBY to ale yeast and wine yeast. By learning the fundamentals of wild yeast, we start in good stead for the following, more complex recipes to come.

YEAST AND HUMANS

It's thought that our relationship with yeasts may have started even before the arrival of *Homo sapiens*, sometime around our last common ancestor with chimpanzees, the CHLCA (Chimpanzee-Human Last Common Ancestor, pronounced "chil-ka"). During this time, a mutation occurred, which meant some individuals could tolerate the effects of alcohol (which, until this point, was a potent toxin that left those who consumed it vulnerable and quickly led to poisoning). This

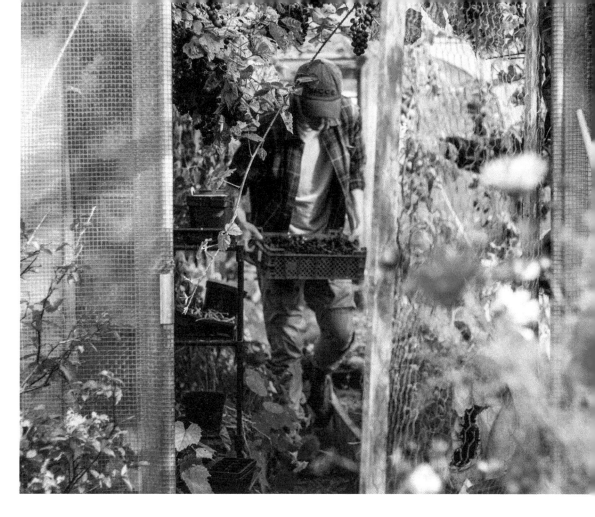

Harvesting grapes for
winemaking from a
solar tunnel in Wales.

new mutation meant ethanol had less impact because it
could be broken down and cleared from the body more
quickly, giving those who carried the mutation access to
a valuable additional food source—fallen fruits that lay
fermenting on the forest floor.

Those who sought out these alcoholic fruits,
potentially by following the thick, heady fragrance of yeast
fermentation (which also attracts butterflies and insects),
will have been rewarded with abundant food that naturally
repelled their competition. Around 10 million years later and
here we are, selecting varieties of fruit for their specific
characteristics that suit alcohol fermentation and mixing
them with yeasts that produce increasingly more prolific
amounts of alcohol.

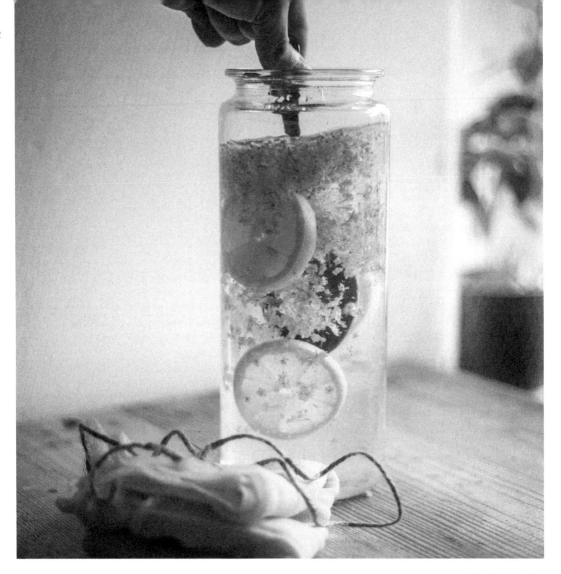

Step 3, mixing the
ingredients into the water.

HERBAL SODA

<0.5 PERCENT ABV

2-liter jar

muslin

string or elastic band

2 × 1-liter bottles

INGREDIENTS

190g sugar, honey,
  or syrup, plus extra
  for carbonation

1.95kg water

1 lemon

about 30g elderflowers
  (fresh or dried)

I was first introduced to wild soda by the work of Pascal Baudar (see further reading, p.218), an author and educator on the subject of wildcrafted foods and fermentation. This 3-day ferment is a quick and delicious way to explore the flavors of wild yeasts in the world around us. With no specialty equipment required, this is a great first step to whet your appetite and costs no more than a bag of sugar.

The basic principle here is sugar to feed the yeast, something acidic, and a breathable lid to prevent fruit flies from getting in. Within these rules, there's room for creativity. While most wines, ciders, and beers celebrate fruits, berries, and grain, for me, sodas are where fragrant ingredients like herbs and edible flowers truly shine. This version showcases elderflower—a gift as spring turns to summer, when a refreshing soda is the perfect treat. See overleaf for my other favorites.

CARBONATION

Natural carbonation often occurs during fermentation, which is why we have to use airlocks or "burp" jars to release pressure (see p.67). But controlled carbonation can transform a finished product. By adding 1–2 teaspoons of additional sugar per 1 liter of a fully fermented beverage when bottling, you can give the yeasts just enough extra food to carbonate most drinks after 2–3 days (depending on temperature).

1. Add the sugar to the jar, then add half the water and stir until dissolved.

2. Wash and cut the lemon into five thick slices and add them in, then stuff in as many elderflowers as you can. The more you add, the stronger the flavor. (Note that elderflower blossom must be cut from the stems, which contain a cyanide-producing chemical that can cause illness.)

3. Finally, top up the jar with the rest of the water, making sure none of the ingredients float above the surface. You can either rely on having packed them in tightly enough, or add a cap to keep them submerged.

4. Attach the muslin to the top using the string or elastic band and leave it on your fermentation shelf for 3 days.

5. After 3 days, pass the soda through a fine-mesh sieve to remove the solid ingredients and divide between two 1-liter bottles with 1–2 teaspoons additional sugar per liter for carbonation.

6. Leave at room temperature for 1–2 days to allow pressure to build, then put in the fridge for a day to chill before serving. They will keep for up to 3 days in the fridge.

HERBAL SODA VARIATIONS

My herbal soda recipe (see pp.122–123) is flavored with elderflower (the exact measurements of which rely on how much you can cram into the jar), but you can try swapping out the elderflower for a herb, or mixing different herbs, fruits, berries, or flowers. See the following recipes for some of my favorites.

LEMON VERBENA

This recipe tastes of lemonade and sherbet. Harvest as much fresh verbena as you can fit in the jar, add slices of fresh lemon, and follow the same steps as the elderflower recipe. You might have trouble keeping the tiny blossoms from floating. If so, simply stir the drink twice a day instead.

ROSE PETAL AND ORANGE

Rose petals are beautifully fragrant as an ingredient in herbal soda, but they are highly sensitive to heat. To help extract as much flavor as possible, I'd recommend using an immersion blender to break up the petals in the soda before adding five slices of orange and fermenting as usual. By day 3, the petals will have browned somewhat, but the drink will take on an amazing color depending on the variety used.

LEMON BALM AND FRESH MINT

Always use a slice of lemon or lime to make the drink acidic and safe. This version produces a beautifully dry, ginlike beverage when served uncarbonated (by omitting the sugar in step 5). By using the stems of the herbs, too, you'll get a more tannic, dry flavor.

MAGNOLIA BLOSSOM

One of the first blossoms of the year, magnolia should be foraged when the buds are still almost closed. They have a sweet floral fragrance, a gingery spice, and an earthy undertone. Remove the gray outer layer and fill the jar with the whole flower. Mash or blend, then leave to macerate and infuse.

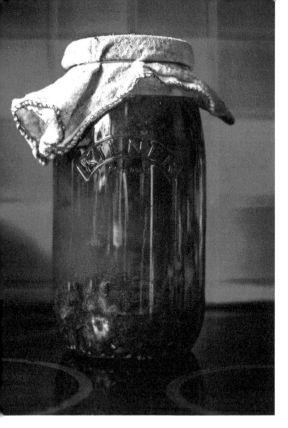

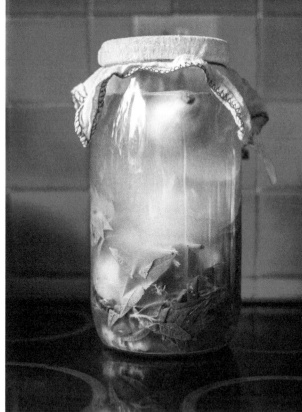

GRAPE, LEMON, AND GINGER ROOT

Fiery and very active, this ferment will burst into life if kept at roughly 77°F (25°C). It is a refreshing spin on grape juice, which also infuses nicely with any additional citrus peels you might have left over. Use half grape juice (from crushed grapes) and half water, with as much ginger as you like. (I crush the ginger in the jar with a rolling pin.) The process will leach the fragrant oils from the peel and create an incredibly refreshing drink. If you like it, you should also try kumquat.

CHERRY BLOSSOM

Another to try with lemon or orange, cherry blossom herbal soda is also incredible with plum, meadowsweet, or apricot blossom. It is deeply perfumed and thick with fragrance.

FRESH NETTLE AND BERGAMOT

Full of iron and minerals, and with a peppery kick and a hint of spinach, fresh nettle needs lemon to liven it up and bring it a much-needed refreshing finish. If you can find it, fresh bergamot works beautifully with nettle.

125

YEAST

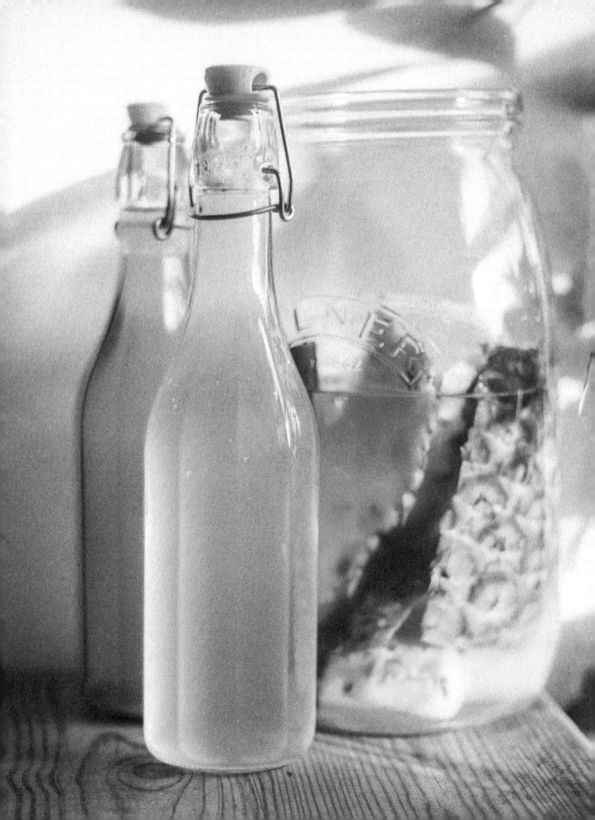

TEPACHE

1–2 PERCENT ABV

EQUIPMENT

3-liter jar

large muslin

string

2 × 1-liter bottles

INGREDIENTS

200g panela

2kg water

1 cinnamon stick

peel and core of
2 pineapples

Tepache, which comes from Mexico, or *aluá*, a similar drink in Brazil, is traditionally made with corn or pineapple peel and core in an elegant example of frugality creating something truly delicious. The versatility of tepache makes it perfect for every season and location.

1. Begin by dissolving the panela in the water in a large, clean pan with the cinnamon. You can warm the water to speed this up, but make sure it cools to below 86°F (30°C) before the next step.

2. Once cool enough, pour it into the jar, add the peel and core of the pineapples, and cover with a large muslin cloth. Tie the muslin in place with string and leave it for 2 days, opening to stir daily.

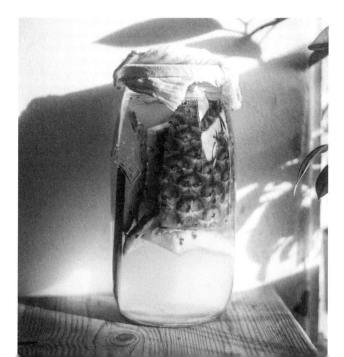

Left Tepache, fermenting on day 2.

Opposite Tepache, bottled and ready to carbonate before refrigerating.

3. After 2 days, remove the muslin and check on the tepache. There should be visible froth around the fruit on the surface; if not, then chances are it isn't warm enough. To kick-start the fermentation again, stir the ingredients well, enough to make a whirlpool in the liquid, then return the cloth and move all of it somewhere warm, such as a linen closet.

4. Once frothy, remove the pineapple and cinnamon, transfer to bottles, and chill for a day. You can cut any edible pineapple into chunks and freeze to use instead of ice to serve. Keep for up to a week in the fridge.

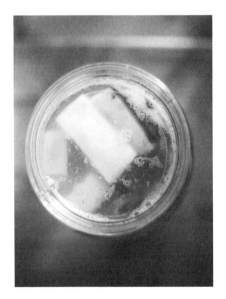

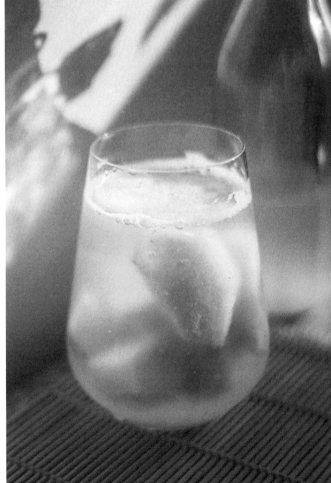

Above Signs of froth appearing on the surface.

Right Carbonated and chilled tepache with frozen pineapple.

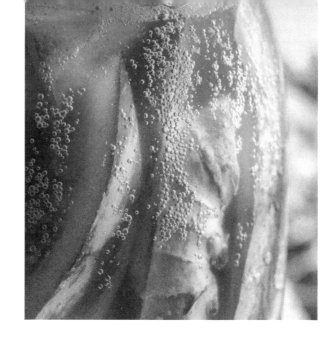

Melon rind with lime tepache is clean, sweet, and refreshing in the heat of the summer. Sometimes I include a piece of ginger root for a gentle warmth.

TEPACHE VARIATIONS

FERMENTER'S NOTE

This drink is traditionally sweetened with panela, known in Mexico as piloncillo. It is made from dried sugar cane juice, and the unrefined sugars provide a rich depth of flavor. If you can't find panela, use raw coconut sugar.

Thanks to the yeast living on the outside of fruit, tepache can be made from almost any ingredient you can get your hands on. Here are some of my favorites.

MELON RIND WITH LIME AND FIG LEAF

This is probably the most refreshing tepache I've ever made; make sure to reserve some melon flesh to freeze instead of ice when serving. If you want to experience something really special, pick young fig leaves and add them to the ferment. These vivid green leaves taste of vanilla and coconut and complement the melon beautifully. The lime is essential for its acidity.

ORANGE PEEL

Save just a few oranges' worth of peel and add to the tepache at the start of the recipe, along with two fresh slices of orange for good measure. Once this ferment kicks into action, it tastes like one of those amazing 1990s ice pops (full of E numbers and probably banned now).

STRAWBERRY AND LEMON

Hull and halve the strawberries and use a floral honey or raw cane sugar to feed this fermentation. Add a slice of lemon, then cover and age as normal. This pink and delicious drink tastes of pure strawberry extract with a powerful aroma reminiscent of the strawberry crème in fancy chocolates.

GINGER BUG

1–2 PERCENT ABV

Ginger is alive with microbes, and I often include it in lacto fermentation to help kick-start the process. Taking the techniques of tepache (see pp.127–129), ginger bug or wild fruit starter is a technique for cultivating wild yeasts and directing them safely toward more specialized alcohol production. The beauty of a ginger bug is that it works with regular store-bought ginger at any time of the year and can be used to further inoculate fruit wines, country wines, beer, and ginger beer. Learning how to make this will set you up in good stead for the yeast-based techniques in this chapter. Think of an established ginger bug as similar to a sourdough starter for lightly alcoholic, sparkling drinks.

Below Step 1, adding ingredients to the jar.

Below right Step 4, the liquid is cloudy with yeast.

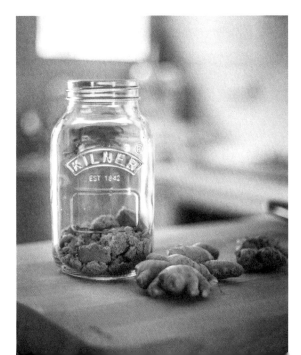

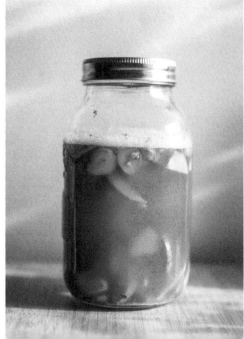

750ml jar with a lid

muslin

string or elastic
band

INGREDIENTS

50g sugar

200g ginger root,
roughly chopped
(no need to peel)

500g water

WILD FRUIT OR
BERRY STARTER

*The exact same method
as outlined above can be
used to harvest microbes
from fruit and berries in
our gardens, hedges, and
woodlands. When foraging,
it's very important to know
what you're picking, and
harvest only ripe,
undamaged ingredients.
Avoid roadside hedges, as
these are often subject to
pollutants from traffic.*

*Once made, the discarded
berries can be used to make
coulis or blended with any
spare starter liquid and dried
into fruit leather, which is
tart or sweet, depending
on how long you've aged
it for (and can complement
both savory and sweet
culinary applications).*

1. Add the sugar to the jar, along with the chopped ginger root and water. Fasten the lid securely, then shake until the sugar is dissolved.

2. Remove the lid and replace it with the muslin. Secure the muslin with string or an elastic band. Put the jar somewhere warm (roughly 77°F/25°C) and stir daily to stop mold growth on the surface.

3. After 3–4 days, the liquid should be alive with bubbles and smell sweet and yeasty.

4. After a week, the ginger bug should be in full swing and ready to use to inoculate a larger batch of alcohol (see ginger beer, p.132).

5. It is possible to keep your ginger bug indefinitely at room temperature by throwing half away and topping it up with more sugar, water, and fresh ginger every so often. However, given how easy it is to make one, I usually start a new one each time.

FERMENTER'S NOTE

*The leftover ginger can
be used to infuse gin,
cooked into jams and
preserves, or thrown on
the compost heap.*

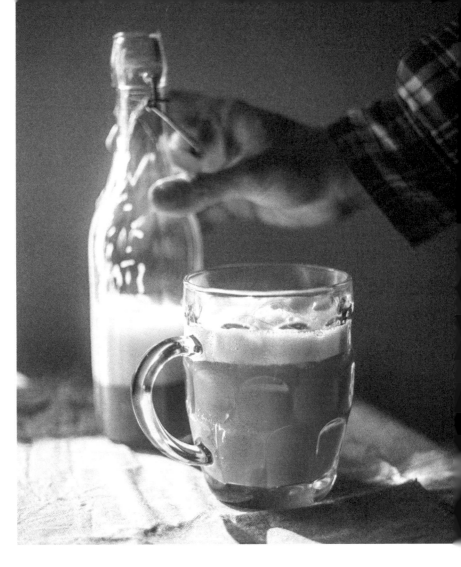

A lively, carbonated ginger beer is a beautiful thing.

GINGER BEER

1–2 PERCENT ABV

FERMENTER'S NOTE

Timings for carbonation can vary depending on the ambient temperature at which you fermented your ginger beer. If you're new to this and worry about exploding bottles and sticky messes, put some of your ginger beer in a plastic bottle and store it along with the glass bottles—you can give it a squeeze to get a feel for how much pressure has built up.

fermentation vessel
with airlock and lid

4 × 1-liter bottles

INGREDIENTS

300g ginger root,
roughly chopped
(no need to peel)

350g sugar or honey

3kg water

500ml active ginger
bug (see pp.130–131)

aromatics, such as
cinnamon sticks or
star anise (optional)

Below Step 1, making
a sweet ginger tea.

Below right Step 2,
inoculating the cooled
tea with an active
ginger bug.

To turn your established ginger bug (see pp.130–131) into
ginger beer, use it to inoculate sweet ginger tea (maximum
scale should be nine times that of your ginger bug). For
additional flavor, feed the ginger beer with unrefined sugar or
honey and include aromatics like cinnamon sticks and star
anise, lightly singed.

1. Add the ginger, sugar, and water to a saucepan with any
   aromatics, and bring to a boil. Simmer for 5 minutes, then
   let it cool completely before removing the ginger.

2. Strain out and discard the old ginger from the active
   ginger bug, then add the ginger bug to the sweet ginger
   tea. Pour the mixture into the sanitized bottles through a
   fine-mesh sieve. Fasten the lid and ferment for 4 days
   at 68°F (20°C).

3. After 4 days, transfer to the fridge and chill for 1 day
   to carbonate (see Fermenter's Note) for a refreshing,
   sparkling ginger beer. Keep for up to 3–4 days in the
   fridge. As this drink is alive with microbes at the time
   it's drunk, I'd advise not drinking too much at once
   (a glass a day is fine).

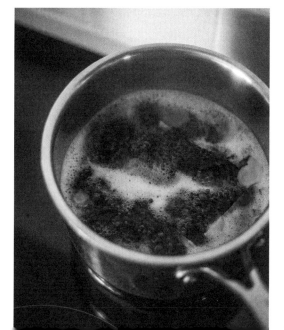

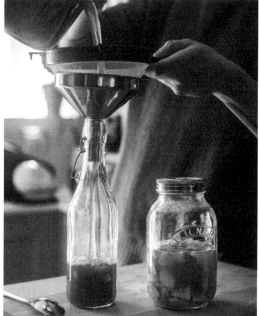

Kombucha has become wildly popular. Originating in China, it is commonly made with an infusion of black tea and sugar. Unlike the previous yeast recipes, kombucha is a continuous fermentation, with a symbiosis between bacteria and yeast (called a SCOBY) at its heart. Famous for this jellyfishlike floating blob of cellulose, nothing says "crazy alchemist" more than a jar of kombucha bubbling away in your kitchen.

The symbiosis of kombucha means the drink will never exceed more than 1–2 percent ABV unless bottled for a long period. This is because the yeast cannot convert sugar to ethanol faster than the bacteria can convert ethanol to acid. For this reason, overly aged kombucha makes a great vinegar substitute, which is ready sooner than regular alcohol and vinegar fermentation.

There are two approaches to kombucha. The first is to brew a batch, then add additional flavors and aromatics at the bottling stage to push the drink into new and exciting infusions. The second is to infuse the additional ingredients up front, then filter the liquid and introduce the SCOBY (see p.136) and ferment the flavors all together. The first method works well if you don't have much storage space, but I prefer the flavors from the second method. However, the cellulose raft or zoogleal mat (a product of the microbial population) picks up flavors, too. So if you've made a batch of bilberry kombucha, you won't want to use the same raft for the following batch of mint kombucha, as it will muddy the flavors. The upside to this is you'll end up with a living library of kombucha flavors; the downside is needing much more storage space to house them all.

Unlike the overly sour home-brewed kombucha of old, and most overly produced commercial kombucha in stores, the following recipes strive for the balance and complexity you'd expect from a well-crafted country wine. Kombucha can be made from almost any lightly sweetened liquid.

KOMBUCHA

0.5–2 PERCENT ABV

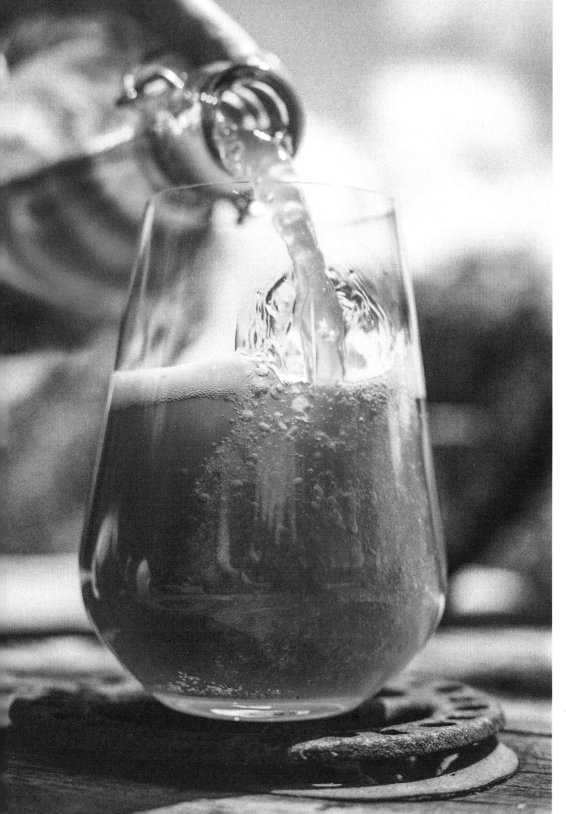

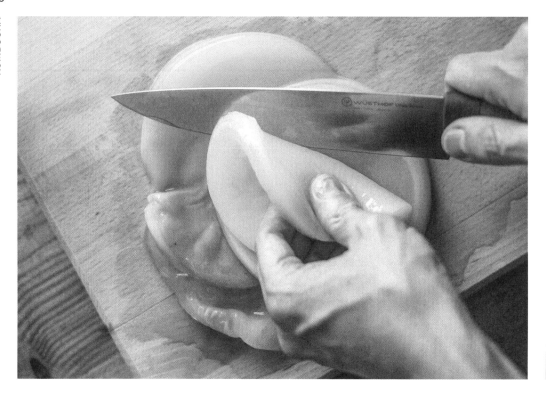

SCOBY

Unlike the other ferments so far, kombucha requires a specific starter to get going. The symbiotic culture of yeast and bacteria living in the liquid form a cellulose raft. This raft will arrive in a small container with some mature kombucha liquid; this is your SCOBY. If you know someone who makes kombucha, then you can ask them for a SCOBY. Or you can buy them online from any good fermentation store.

FEEDING THE SCOBY

You'll need to make 2–3 batches of sweet tea to revive the SCOBY before using it in a kombucha recipe (see pp.139–142). As soon as you can, make a batch of sweet tea that's nine times the weight of the SCOBY and about 10°Bx (10 percent sugar). Let it cool, then add the SCOBY. (This includes the liquid.) Ferment in a sanitized container with a breathable lid for 1 week at 77°F (25°C), then repeat the process, transferring the SCOBY each time.

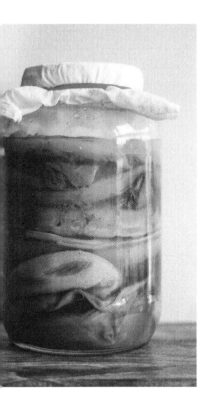

Above left Dividing a cellulose mat that has grown too big.

Above A SCOBY hotel in 20 percent sugar solution.

USING A SCOBY IN THE RECIPES

The microbial community of kombucha lives throughout the liquid and raft, but most people refer to the raft alone as the SCOBY. For the purpose of the following recipes, I will refer to the raft as the SCOBY and list the raw, mature kombucha separately to make sure the correct measurements are followed and avoid confusion.

SCOBY STORAGE

As you make multiple batches of kombucha, you'll not only notice that your raft grows over time, but that it can multiply in layers, with the young, fresh raft appearing at the surface of the liquid, pushing the older, darker-colored one down below. To maintain control over the speed and flavor of your kombucha, it's important to manage how much raft is added to fresh brews, so you may need to intervene and cut it down to a manageable size. This can be done with a clean, sharp knife, as it's surprisingly tough.

You can store the spare raft in what's commonly called a SCOBY hotel, a plain sugar syrup where the SCOBY is held in stasis until you need it to make more kombucha. By upping the amount of sugar to 20 percent and chilling the vessel, you can slow the activity right down. It will still need a breathable lid and fresh food in the form of more sugar syrup every 6 weeks or so. Most importantly, try not to forget about it and let the top dry out.

SHARING YOUR SCOBY

Transporting and sharing your SCOBY with friends is much easier than you might think. Lift the cellulose raft from the kombucha and place it on a clean plate. Take a sharp knife and cut a piece free. This can be done horizontally between the layers or vertically through them. You won't hurt or damage the raft. Place the spare part in a clean lunch box or jar with enough mature kombucha liquid (preferably recently fed) to cover it and fasten with an airtight lid. Remember, the SCOBY needs oxygen, so encourage your friend to prepare its new home ASAP.

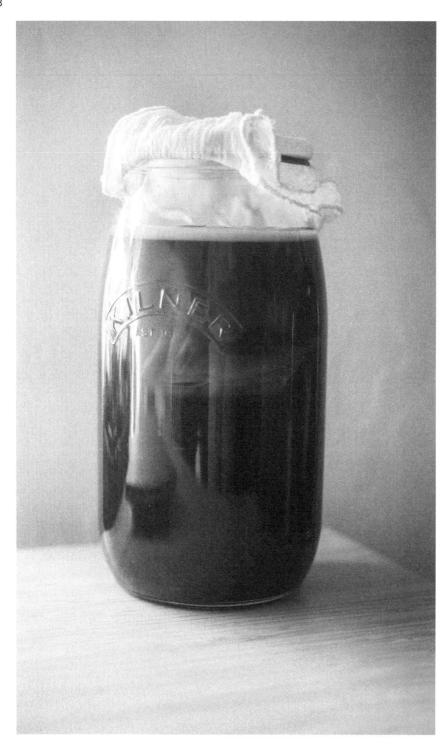

Step 3, after 5–7
days, the SCOBY has
developed a new layer
of cellulose at the
liquid's surface.

BLACK TEA KOMBUCHA

EQUIPMENT

2.5-liter jar

muslin

string

3 × 750ml bottles

INGREDIENTS

2kg water

8 tbsp black tea (made
from 5 tea bags)

220g raw cane sugar

220g mature kombucha
(kombucha that has been
fermented and tastes sour)

a SCOBY (see box, p.137)

COOKING
WITH FERMENTS

VINEGAR SUBSTITUTE
AND GLAZE

If you overferment kombucha into a
potent sour beast, all is not lost. By
gently reducing it for a few hours until
it reaches the consistency of a glaze,
you can create a vinegar substitute.
It pairs nicely with caramel sauce;
can be used as a glaze for meats
or mushrooms; makes a wonderful
partner for dipping oil with bread;
and gives depth and acidity to soups,
stews, and sauces.

DRINKING VINEGAR

Use overly soured kombucha as a
cordial shot in sparkling water with
ice and flavor with fresh herbs.

What most people think of as original kombucha, black tea
kombucha boasts strong malty, astringent tannic flavors
with fermented tang. This version aims to capture the
kombucha before it becomes too sour, relying on the
residual sweetness and mild acidity to balance the tea's
bitterness without overpowering its other characteristics.

1. Begin by heating 500g water with the tea and sugar.
   Stir gently to infuse and dissolve for 5 minutes, then
   remove the teabags (or filter it through muslin if you
   have used leaves) and add the remaining cold water.
   This will lower the temperature enough not to kill the
   SCOBY when added.

2. Pour the entire mixture into the jar and add the mature
   kombucha and raft. The addition of mature kombucha
   lowers the pH enough to protect the fresh batch from
   the takeover of pathogenic microbes that can't
   tolerate the acidity or competition from thriving
   kombucha. Secure a piece of muslin over the top
   with string.

3. Leave it somewhere warmer than room temperature,
   ideally 77–86°F (25–30°C), to ferment for 5–7 days.
   During this time, keep an eye on the raft. They tend to
   float and the top can dry out. If it does, this could lead to
   unwanted mold growth, so make sure to baste it with
   kombucha every now and again.

4. Start tasting it after day 5. Once the kombucha has
   reached a pleasant acidity, it is ready to bottle. To do so,
   remove the raft and reserve 250g of the mature liquid.
   Filter the rest into bottles with 1 teaspoon sugar per 750ml
   bottle for extra fizz.

5. Store the bottles for 1–2 days at room temperature, then
   refrigerate for 2–3 days to allow a pleasant carbonation
   to build up. Store in a fridge for up to 3 months.

KOMBUCHA VARIATIONS

For these recipes, follow the step-by-step instructions for the black tea kombucha (see p.139) and simply swap out the tea for the ingredient of your choice. I've listed whether you should use a gentle heat or cold (overnight) infusion prior to adding sugar and inoculating with 10 percent mature kombucha and a SCOBY (see box, p.137). Besides the hops, which I'd recommend not using more than 30g, the other recipes are completely up to you. If you love rose, the more you can cram in, the better. Really into mint? Pack it full. And why not use peppermint and spearmint? Have fun!

HOPS AND CRYSTAL MALT KOMBUCHA

Fruity, malted, and funky. Simmer the hops and malt at 149°F (65°C) for 1 hour, then filter and dissolve the sugar. Let cool to 86°F (30°C), then inoculate with 10 percent mature kombucha and a SCOBY (see box, p.137). Ferment as the black tea kombucha, or age for 3 weeks to create a hoppy, sour vinegar that brings depth to savory, meaty casseroles.

ROSE KOMBUCHA

Floral and perfumed. Remove the petals from fragrant roses and pulse in a food processor a few times in cold water. Cover and infuse for 12–24 hours somewhere chilled, then filter to remove the petals the next day. Add and dissolve the sugar, inoculate with 10 percent mature kombucha and a SCOBY (see box, p.137), and continue as outlined in the black tea kombucha recipe. Taste after 5 days to catch some remaining sweetness that complements the rose.

MINT KOMBUCHA

Mint suits both a hot and a cold infusion, offering different flavors for each. Moroccan mint and black mint are particularly delicious as kombucha, but explore other varieties. Infuse for 24 hours in cold water, or plunge into freshly boiled water and soak until cold. Dissolve the sugar, inoculate with 10 percent mature kombucha and a SCOBY (see box, p.137), and continue as the black tea kombucha.

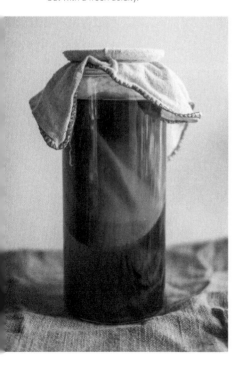

Malt kombucha, which is distinctly beerlike, but with a fresh acidity.

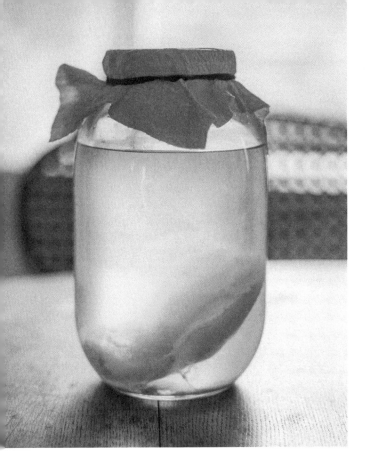

Orange kombucha, from the recipe below.

FIG LEAF KOMBUCHA

A grassy vanilla or coconut aroma. Pick young fig leaves and soak in hot water for an hour, then filter and dissolve the sugar. Inoculate with 10 percent mature kombucha and a SCOBY (see box, p.137) and ferment as outlined in the black tea kombucha recipe. Once made, this kombucha is perfectly suited for using in custards, sorbet, and ice cream.

ORANGE KOMBUCHA

Pure orange flavor as you've never experienced it before (which also complements additions of ginger root and rose petals). Use orange flesh and peel, but do not use waxed fruit, and wash first. Dissolve the sugar in hot water, then add the orange and peel while warm to extract fragrant oils from the skin. Let cool, then filter and inoculate with 10 percent mature kombucha and a SCOBY (see box, p.137). This is great soured and added to desserts or frozen as granita.

141

HONEY KOMBUCHA

This recipe relies on the quality of honey you use. In Wales, I'm lucky enough to have access to heather honey, apple blossom honey, and hedgerow honey, which offer a range of floral delights. Most honey is 82 percent sugar, so dissolve an additional 22 percent honey to bring the sugar level up to the correct amount to ferment. (For example, the black tea kombucha recipe uses 220g of sugar but would require 268g of honey to make the equivalent amount of sugar.) Dissolve it in hot water and infuse with tea, then inoculate with 10 percent mature kombucha and a SCOBY (see box, p.137). Continue as written in the black tea kombucha recipe.

FRUIT SYRUPS

You can turn any fruit or berries into a syrup to feed kombucha, but you'll have to adjust the amount of sugar you add to compensate for the sugar that is already present in the ingredients. Aim for a Brix reading of 10–12°Bx, but don't worry if it's a little higher or lower. Juice the ingredients and pass the liquid through a cloth or fine-mesh sieve and test the Brix level using a refractometer (see p.117), then add more sugar to bring the overall amount needed to the right level. For berries that are high in pectin, freeze and thaw them first for a cleaner mouthfeel to the final kombucha.

KOMBUCHA CREAM

FERMENTER'S NOTE

You can add the following flavorings to your kombucha cream, folding them inin step 4:
- *½ tsp vanilla paste*
- *½ tsp rose water*
- *fruits (edible pieces, zest, and juice)*
- *a handful of berries (including coulis and jams)*

Once you've made kombucha, you not only have a delicious drink and cooking liquid at your disposal, but also a means to make a sour cream with the infusion of whatever flavor kombucha you've made. This is a much faster ferment than kombucha itself and leaves you with a crème-fraîche-like ingredient that's gorgeous in rice pudding, crème Anglaise, and white sauces. The fragrance of the kombucha infuses nicely with the fat of the cream. My favorite use is frozen, as it reminds me of a cheap ice pop I used to have as a kid (only a little more sophisticated).

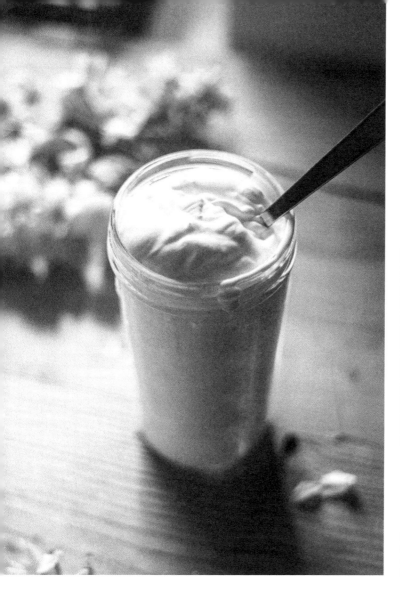

KOMBUCHA ICE CREAM

Whip the kombucha cream, as step 4, then pour into silicone molds and freeze overnight.

KOMBUCHA GRANITA

Add fragrant ingredients like edible flower petals, citrus peel, blossom water, bitter almond, or pistachio to whipped kombucha cream (or even regular kombucha, see orange kombucha, p.141). Sweeten to taste and freeze it. Once an hour, rake the mixture with a fork and return it to the freezer. After 4 hours, the granita is ready.

Kombucha cream makes an excellent alternative to any recipe that calls for regular cream, offering additional tang.

EQUIPMENT

muslin

string

INGREDIENTS

500ml heavy cream

50ml kombucha

30g honey or sugar

1. Put the cream in a bowl, add the kombucha, and mix.

2. Cover with muslin secured with string and leave to ferment at 68°F (20°C) for 24–36 hours.

3. After this stage, chill in the fridge for at least 4 hours.

4. Add the honey or sugar. If you would like it whipped, gently whip for 2–3 minutes until stiff. Store in the fridge for up to 3 days (or make into ice cream, see above).

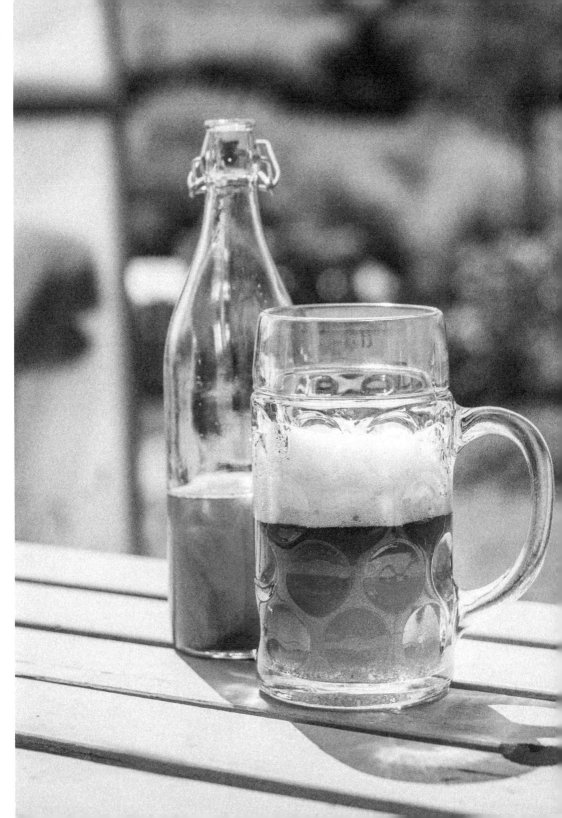

OAT BEER

5-6 PERCENT ABV

My first steps into the world of home-brewed alcohol were with a good friend, Ben Lavery, many, many years ago. He grew up brewing beer with his dad, but having moved away from home, he and I set out on our first independent voyage with one goal in mind: to attempt to replicate a famous Welsh beer called Butty Bach (meaning "little friend") from the Wye Valley Brewery. What we loved about Butty Bach was its creaminess, and we had a hunch we knew how it was done—oats.

You can think of the beer-making process as an extension of kombucha making. In short, a tealike infusion of ingredients that are then sweetened with sugar and offered up to yeast for a number of months. Unlike kombucha, beer isn't granted access to oxygen, stopping bacteria from souring it. Instead, the alcohol level continues to build.

Luckily for me, Ben is a beer fanatic, but also has a fondness for typewriters. So I still have a hand-typed copy of the original recipe framed, which I've written up below. He named it Cwrw Butty Dda (said "koo-roo butty tha"), which is Welsh for "Beer of Good Friends." Tradition dictates that you invite a friend or two over to help with the preparation, ideally in a well-ventilated room, as it'll produce a lot of steam. And of course, you have to share the finished beer with said friends, too.

A beer I make with (and for) my friends, which has never left Wales until now.

EQUIPMENT

large pan or stock
pot (6 imperial
gallons)

large straining bag

fermentation bin

airlock

2 muslin bags

hydrometer

25 × 750ml bottles

siphon pump

INGREDIENTS

5 (imperial) gallons
water

3kg pale malt,
crushed (Maris
Otter is preferable)

500g crystal malt,
crushed

75g goldings hops

150g rolled oats

500g demerara
sugar, plus extra
for bottling

1 sachet beer (ale)
yeast

1. Mashing: Put the water in the large stock pot and heat to 149°F (65°C), then add the pale and crystal malts. Infuse for 3 hours over very low heat, checking back from time to time to ensure that the temperature of 149°F (65°C) is maintained.

2. Sparging: Strain and discard the solids from the sweet wort (the infused liquid), then pass the liquid through the large straining bag three times until it is completely clear. On the final strain, collect the liquid (wort) in the fermentation bin. Clean and dry the large pan.

3. Boiling: Bring the wort back to the heat in the clean, dry pan and top it back up to 5 gallons, if necessary. Bring to a boil and add 50g hops and 100g oats to one of the muslin bags. Add them to the boiling wort and simmer for 1 hour 30 minutes, stirring occasionally.

4. Add the remaining hops and oats in the second bag and continue to boil for another 15 minutes. During this 15 minutes, make sure the fermentation bin is cleaned and sanitized, then add the sugar.

5. Pour the wort into the fermentation bin and stir to dissolve the sugar. Remove the muslin bags.

6. Fermenting: Allow the wort to cool to 64–68°F (18–20°C), then take a gravity reading using a hydrometer (see p.118). Stir in the yeast and secure the lid with an airlock.

7. For the first 3 days, remove any scum that forms on the surface.

8. On day 6, take another gravity reading on a hydrometer (see p.118).

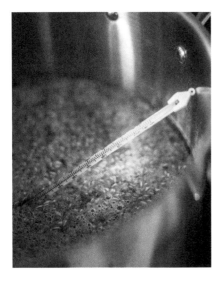

Step 1, mashing,
carefully monitoring
the temperature as
the malts infuse.

9. On day 8, take another reading. If the gravity is stable, prepare for bottling. If not, wait another few days and repeat. If you lack a hydrometer, wait 10 days from adding the yeast before bottling.

10. Bottling: Add 1 teaspoon of sugar to each of the sanitized bottles, then siphon the wort into each bottle, taking care not to disturb the sediment at the bottom of the fermentation bin. Cap each bottle, upend, and shake to dissolve the sugar. Store in a cool place for 3 weeks.

11. You can then store it for up to 1 year in the fridge, but drink at just below room temperature. Once opened, store in the fridge and drink within 3 days of opening.

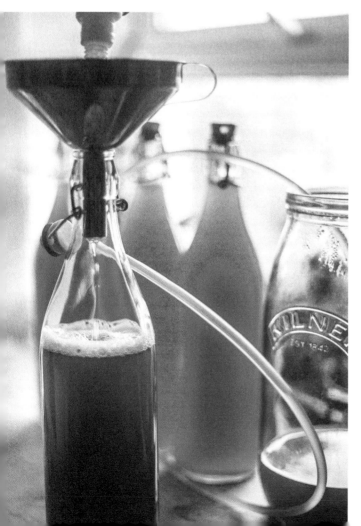

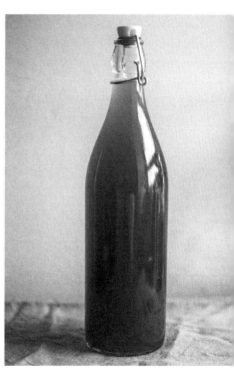

Above Oat beer aged for 3 weeks.

Left Step 10, bottling is best done with the fermentation vessel elevated above the bottle.

147

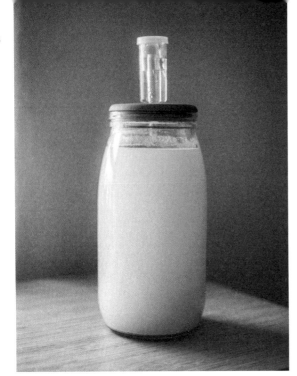

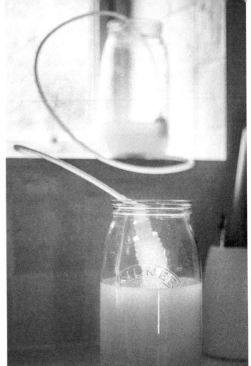

Above left Steps 4–5: the mead has slowed down but is still cloudy with yeast and bubbling a little.

Above The first racking: transferring the mead to another vessel to leave behind the sediment.

MEAD

11 PERCENT ABV

It's only fitting that I include a mead recipe in this book, as mead is a drink I fell in love with when I moved to Wales, where it has a long history. It is the Welsh who wrote about drinking sparkling honey wine from a hollowed-out horn (in the poem "Kanu y med" by Taliesin, 550 CE). Another poem called "Y Gododdin by Aneirin," described going to battle drunk on mead: "Their high spirits lessened their life span." The Welsh word for getting drunk is even "meddwi" (pronounced meth-we), and directly translates as "meaded."

While the recipe I decided to include is definitely a modern take on that of old (which wasn't very alcoholic and tasted very yeasty), it's still deliciously floral and dry and follows a very similar technique. In mead-making, the quality of the honey you use makes all the difference. I am lucky enough to know beekeepers in my area who tend to some hives of the Welsh Black Honeybee, which it is said is the only bee that flies during rain. You can also make a

EQUIPMENT

3.5-liter jar

hydrometer

airlock

siphon pump

bottles with corks

INGREDIENTS

2.4kg water

600g raw honey,
preferably fresh
and local

white wine yeast or
Champagne yeast

yeast nutrient and
acidity regulator
(optional)

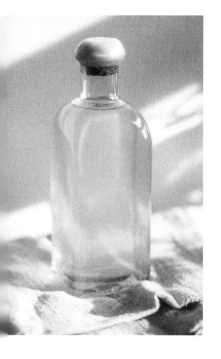

Fully fermented mead,
bottled and sealed with
beeswax.

traditional medicinal version of mead called a metheglin (meddylgyn) by adding aromatic herbs.

Mead can range from a sweet, fruity nectar to a dry, crisp, manzanillalike drink with delicate honey fragrance. It's all about the yeast you use. If you prefer it sweeter, use a dessert wine yeast; if you'd like something dryer, use a white wine or Champagne yeast, as here. Not only will the yeast you use alter the final mead, but it will even change the color and viscosity of the drink.

1. Bring the water to a boil, add to the jar (taking care not to crack the glass with the heat by warming the jar first), and leave to cool a little.

2. Make sure the wax is removed from the raw honey (along with any pieces of bee that might be caught up) and dissolve the honey into the water. To pasteurize the honey, do this while it's still hot. There are qualities to the honey that will be lost, but this also rules out certain bad players. (Alternatively, you can dissolve it into cold water and rely on the production of alcohol and acidity regulator to make it safe.) Allow to cool.

3. Once cooled, take a gravity reading on a hydrometer (see p.118), which should be near 1.080. Add the yeast; yeast nutrient (as per the instructions on the pack), if using; and an acidity regulator for safety, if using, and cover with a lid and airlock.

4. Store above 66°F (19°C) for 2–3 weeks. It should produce lots of carbon dioxide and bubble away.

5. Once activity slows or stops, use a siphon pump to draw some of the liquid and take another gravity reading (which should be between 1.000 and 0.990). Calculate that the ABV is around 11 percent and add the rest into sanitized bottles (taking care not to disturb the sediment at the bottom) and cork them. If the mead isn't quite at the right ABV but all activity seems to have stopped, proceed to bottle.

6. Age in the bottle for a minimum of a month and enjoy at room temperature.

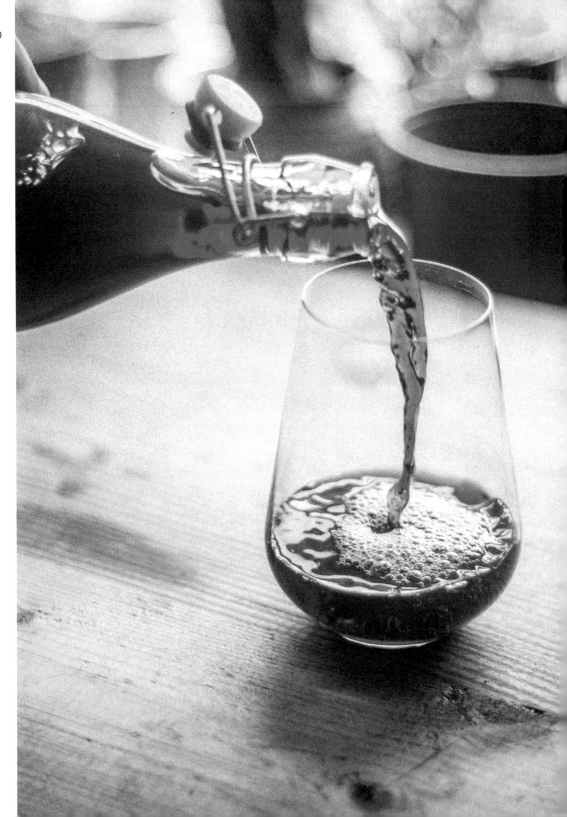

SWEET BLACKCURRANT WINE

9 PERCENT ABV

A classic country wine is made using the wild yeast on the skin of the fruit. While this technique works well most of the time, more often than not, I make a wild alcohol starter (see p.131) a few days prior and use this to inoculate the larger batch. For a more controlled result, you can also use brewer's yeast (either dessert wine or Champagne yeast) and follow the instructions listed on the pack.

Under ideal conditions, yeast will produce 1 percent alcohol per every 18g sugar in 1 liter liquid. This is important to remember, as you can calculate the amount of sugar in your ingredients. Take a measurement of the sugars in your ingredients with a refractometer (see p.117), then figure out if you need to increase it by adding more sugar or decrease it by adding more water. The alcohol content we're aiming for is 5–9 percent: 5 percent is the threshold for safety, but if it goes above 9 percent, it'll be much harder to turn into vinegar at a later date (if that is something you're interested in).

This general process for winemaking works with any fruit or berry and can include aromatic ingredients like rose, magnolia, elderflower, or meadowsweet. You can also use store-bought fruit juices, but double-check the ingredients list. Make sure they're pure fruit juice and make your calculations based on the sugar content listed on the back.

Sweet blackcurrant wine is a ruby-red summer wine, but this process also works wonderfully for strawberry or gooseberry wine.

151

YEAST

EQUIPMENT

refractometer

straining bag

demijohn

airlock

hydrometer

siphon

INGREDIENTS

2kg blackcurrants

4kg water

735g sugar

550ml wild alcohol starter
or dessert wine yeast

yeast nutrient (optional)

1. Prepare the blackcurrants by freezing them for 12 hours to break down the pectin. This will improve the mouthfeel of the finished wine.

2. After 12 hours, bring the water to a boil, then set aside to cool while you remove any woody parts or spoiled currants. Add them to a large mixing bowl with the water once it has cooled, then cover the container with a dish towel and leave it somewhere cool (below 59°F/15°C) to macerate overnight.

3. The next day, either crush by hand (which takes time but is quite satisfying) or pulse them a few times in a food processor to break them up and release their juice. Add the sugar and stir until dissolved. (For accuracy, you can use a refractometer [see p.117] to measure the natural sugars of the blackcurrants, which is 135g in the whole 2kg, then add enough sugar to bring the juice up to a wine fermentation range.) Cover and return to the same location for another 24 hours.

4. Inoculate with the yeast and leave to ferment in the bowl for 48 hours, stirring once a day. Make sure to cover with a dish towel again to prevent fruit flies from getting in.

Below Step 2, infusing frozen blackcurrants in prepared water.

Below right Step 3, pulsed blackcurrants.

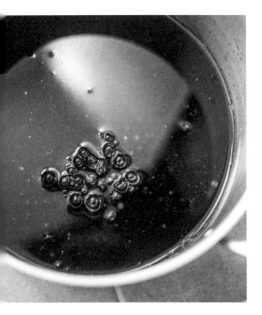

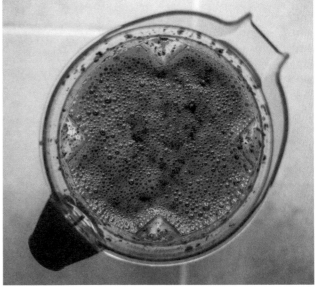

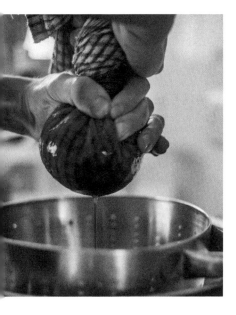
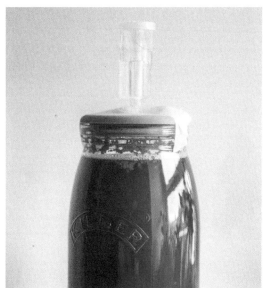

Above Step 5, filter the wine to remove the pulp.

Above right Step 6, the wine was so active that the lid had to be secured with tape.

5. On day 4, pass the wine through a straining bag and press the remaining juice from the pulp. (You can use the pulp to cook into preserves and desserts.) Take a gravity reading using a hydrometer (see p.118) of the clear liquid and make a note of the result.

6. Move it to a clean demijohn for secondary fermentation. Fit the demijohn with an airlock and leave it somewhere 68–77°F (20–25°C), out of direct sunlight, for 1–2 weeks.

7. After a few weeks, use the siphon to rack the wine (collect the clear wine from the demijohn and leave the sediment behind at the bottom).

8. Pour the clear wine into a fresh jar and fit with another airlock. Continue to age the wine for 6 months before bottling it (during which time you may wish to rack it again to remove more sediment).

9. When there is no sign of activity, take a gravity reading and check the alcohol content of the wine. Try a little and sweeten to taste, then bottle in sanitized bottles, cork, and store somewhere cool and out of direct sunlight. The wine is ready to drink whenever you like and should slowly develop different characteristics with time.

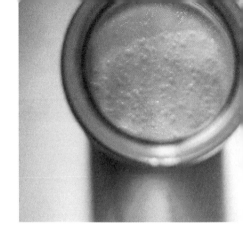

VINEGAR

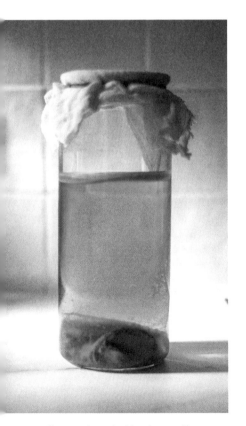

Homemade apple cider vinegar with vinegar mothers gathered at the bottom.

Thanks to the return of an old friend, acetic acid bacteria (AAB, see p.65), any alcohol can be turned into a deliciously tart vinegar to be used for salad dressings, dipping breads, cooking, or as a drinking vinegar. Vinegar is one of the oldest ways to add an acidic kick to food and complements even not-so-obvious pairings like strawberries, ice cream, and desserts. It also plays a crucial role in one of the first preserving techniques I was shown in kitchens: pickling.

If you've gone to the effort of making your own alcohol, then I recommend you reserve some for vinegar-making. But you can also use store-bought alcohols and use the equation below to calculate the potential conversion of ethanol to acid. Note: This is under ideal conditions, so this should be used as guidance and not gospel. Alcohols above 15 percent ABV won't work, as AAB cannot tolerate such a hostile environment. To counter this, cook off the alcohol from a little of the beverage and top it up again with the remaining alcohol, bringing the total ABV down (see Fermenter's Note).

$$\text{Acidity} = \text{ABV} \times 0.8$$

Therefore, if your wine has an alcohol content of 7 percent, multiply this by 0.8, giving us 5.6 percent acidity. Notice this is a percentage of acid in the entire solution and not the same as a pH reading (which is a scale ranging 0–14). In fact, 5.6 percent acidity will display between 2.5–3 pH.

A new vinegar mother forming at the surface (which will soon drop as it ages).

1. First, remove the airlock or bottle cap from your alcohol. The key difference between alcohol and acetic acid fermentation is oxygen. This process can be sped up from the start with an air pump or with daily vigorous stirring.

2. Pour the alcohol into a wide-mouth jar and secure a paper or fabric towel over the top. It's important to change the container or you risk the chance of producing a vinegar mother that ends up stuck in the bottle.

3. If you happen to have some homemade vinegar lying around or a store-bought raw vinegar (often labeled as "with mother"), then inoculate the alcohol with up to 10 percent of this. Much like the kombucha process, this will introduce a healthy population of bacteria that hedges your bets (and lowers the pH, which helps protect the ferment from spoilage). If you don't have any, you can simply leave the alcohol to spontaneously ferment, which it will, as long as the ABV is at or below 13 percent.

4. This process can take anywhere from a few weeks for a light, fruity vinegar, to a few months for something more punchy and sour. The time also varies depending on temperature and time of year. Vinegars produce zoogleal mats like kombucha, but these often sink to the bottom of a jar instead of floating. If one does happen to get stuck at the surface, use a clean spoon to push it down, or it might dry and go moldy. If you happen to make one of these, you can use it to inoculate future vinegars in the same fashion as kombucha making.

FERMENTER'S NOTE

If making vinegar from a drink with higher levels of ethanol, you can either water it down (which will also dilute the flavor) or cook off the excess alcohol. To do this, make a note of the ABV and set some of the liquid aside. Burn off the ethanol from the remaining liquid, then, once cooled, top up with the reserved liquid to bring the alcohol level back up to 8 percent. Once the ABV is adjusted, follow the previous method as normal.

A vinegar concentrate made from
gooseberry wine, which has been
reduced by two-thirds.

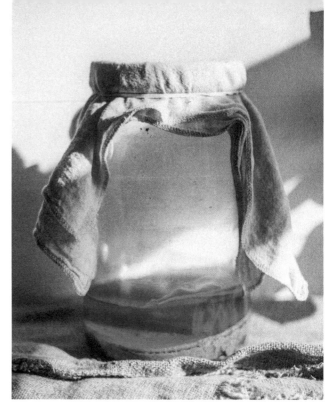

*VI*NEGAR
CONCENTR*ATE*

Turn your vinegar into a clear, concentrated concoction
resembling balsamic richness by forgetting about it. As
vinegar is left to breathe, it will also slowly evaporate and
reduce. While balsamic vinegar is officially reduced in
wooden barrels for a minimum of 12 years, this version
mimics an accelerated process that resembles a similar
fruity richness and can be made from any vinegar.

By leaving it in a jar covered with muslin, once it
reaches full acidity, it becomes shelf stable but continues
to age and reduce. The color darkens as it becomes richer
and beautifully tart. I leave my vinegar concentrate for a
minimum of a year, during which time it reduces by half the
volume. Rack the vinegar into a clean, sanitized bottle,
leaving a small amount of liquid behind to cover the
cellulose mothers. The vinegar reduction can be stored at
room temperature indefinitely and the mothers can be
stored in an airtight container in a fridge for a year until
needed again for another batch.

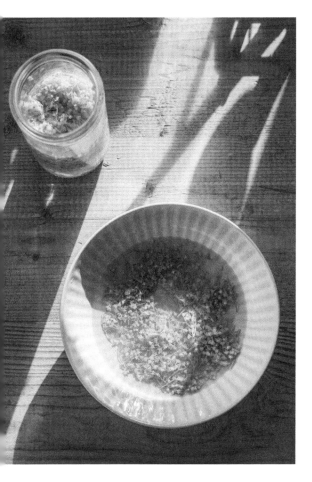

Elderflower, which has been
pickled in homemade vinegar
for 1 year.

PICKLED ELDERFLOWER

Shake 20 fresh elderflower crowns to remove insects and cut the flowers from the stems. Put them in a 700ml jar with 500ml apple cider vinegar, secure the lid so that no air remains in the container, and age in a fridge for at least 6–7 months. The acidity of vinegar will damage metal lids, which in turn will ruin a pickle. Use glass or plastic lids, or cover the pickle with plastic wrap before fastening a metal lid in place.

PICKLING

In pickling, vinegar is mixed 1:1 with water, along with a pinch of salt and sugar to taste, and infused with herbs to produce deliciously sour, crunchy vegetables. To preserve short-lived ingredients outside of their season, I pickle them in pure homemade vinegar, with a pinch of salt and sugar, and store them in a fridge for 6 months minimum.

157

YEAST

The most complex life form you will learn to wield in this book, mold is capable of producing a host of enzymes while simultaneously acting as a facilitator for other microorganisms. For a lot of people, mold, probably more than any other microbe, strikes fear. Often associated with the visible signs of spoilage, we do battle with molds wherever we find them. However, some mold varieties are remarkable, beneficial forms of life.

MOLD

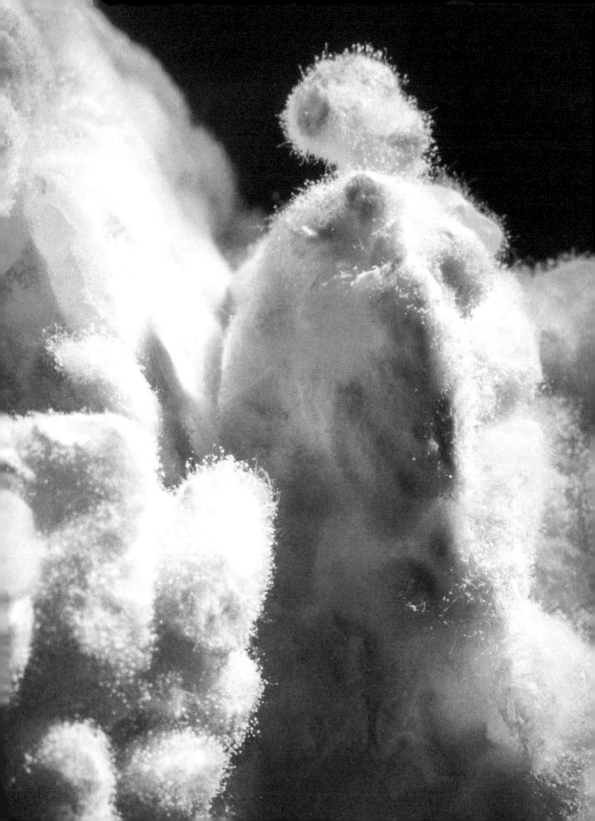

WHAT IS MO*LD*?

Molds fall into the kingdom of fungi, which boasts some of the largest and oldest living organisms on the planet, ranging tens of miles in size and thousands of years in age. And, despite how squeamish some may be, most of us use mold-related products in our day-to-day lives, such as biological detergents, where the "biological" part refers to enzymes that break down stains—enzymes produced by the same mold that gives us soy sauce and miso.

Slime mold, when given a scaled-down map of London with food laid out at what would be each station, grows into a near-perfect replica of the London Underground. Mold growth starts from a single spore with a rootlike structure of multicellular filaments (hyphae) that grow in search of moisture and nutrients to form a mycelial web. In foods like tempeh from Indonesia, this mycelial web is so dense and cottony, it knits the substrate of soybeans or cereal together into a block. The same is true for the characteristic white bloom on Camembert cheese, or veins of blue mold in Stilton, both of which belong to the *Penicillium* genus (*candidum/camemberti* and *roqueforti*), making them cousins of the famous variety discovered by the Scottish physician and microbiologist Sir Alexander Fleming, which produces penicillin, an antibiotic that gives the mold an advantage over its bacterial competition.

The power that mold wields over the other microbes in this book is the sheer breadth and versatility of its enzymes. For the many complex molecules that make up our food, mold has an arsenal of these tiny tools to cleave them apart, increasing bioavailability, and, most importantly, flavors we cannot access alone. It can turn a bean into a rich, fruity, umami miso; turn rice into a sweet liquid drink; and give many cheeses their characteristic punchy aromas and very pleasant flavors.

ASPERGILLUS ORYZAE

A microbe that's big enough to see with the naked eye (just about)—it thrives on substrates like grains.

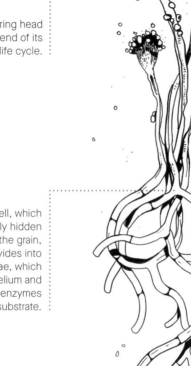

The sporing head at the end of its 48-hour life cycle.

The foot cell, which is usually hidden within the grain, divides into hyphae, which form mycelium and release enzymes into the substrate.

ASPERGILLUS ORYZAE

If a single microorganism could define the cuisine of countless countries, inspire innovation steeped in the tradition of family legacies, and shape an entire continent, *Aspergillus* is the one. It has origins all across East Asia, but it has a special significance in Japan, where it is hailed as the national fungus. It has become globally celebrated thanks to ingredients like miso, jiang, soy sauce, and mirin. All owe their incredible flavor to *A. oryzae*, but so do sake, shochu, meju, rice vinegar, katsuobushi, shio kōji, and amazake, paving the way for its use in culinary adventure.

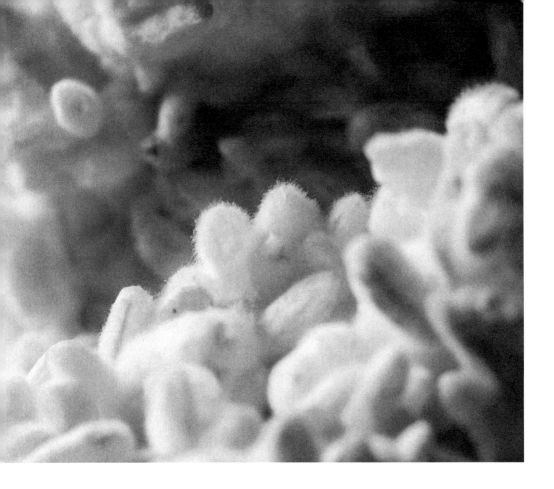

Fluffy white grains of rice covered in *Aspergillus*, caught 30 minutes or so before developing spores.

INTRODUCING KŌJI

When *A. oryzae* spores land on a substrate such as steamed rice, they will produce tiny branching cells (hyphae) that grow to form a network called mycelium. At our scale, the growth of *A. oryzae* develops as a fuzzy exterior that mats the substrate together. At this stage, it becomes what we call kōji—a name given to the combined mold and its substrate— and releases a sweet jasmine aroma before reaching its final stage and producing thin, hairlike stems that release spores for the next generation. This entire process takes just 48 hours, and then you can dry and store the kōji for later use.

My first true face-to-face meeting with it came when I knocked on the door of kōji master Haruko Uchishiba, a Japanese fermenter and supplier living in London. I'm pretty sure she is single-handedly responsible for

Steps must be taken to avoid allowing bacteria and yeast to overrun the mold.

spreading the secret magic of kōji to most of London's top chefs, and they were likely greeted in the same manner, with the excited barking of two very old, very beautiful dogs. Over the following days, I prepared, ate, and even slept beside kōji. We took breaks and ate delicious meals prepared by Haruko, using kōji in both traditional and innovative ways, but it was during an early start one day that Haruko appeared from the kitchen holding two bowls of food that looked a little different. She apologized and explained these weren't for us, but were in fact homemade dog food, loaded with kōji enzymes. In their old age, her dogs had health complications and digestive issues, so she had taken to preparing their meals herself and used kōji to supplement them, producing enzymes and unlocking nutrients the dogs themselves no longer could. I watched in amazement as she lovingly tended to her pets and wondered if the dogs, much like most people who add a dash of soy sauce to their meal or miso to their broth, have any idea of the microbial wonder that makes their food possible.

MULTICELLULAR FERMENTATION

As a mold, *A. oryzae* is the most complex microorganism we will use for fermentation in this book, boasting the greatest versatility in enzymes. Steps must be taken to avoid allowing bacteria and yeast to overrun the mold, as the smaller, more simple life forms can multiply more quickly and take over. But having an understanding of how both bacteria and yeast work from the previous recipes will give you a firm grasp on why certain methods are implemented over the following pages. Welcome to the world of multicellular fermentation.

KŌJI THE FACILITATOR

Foods such as miso, jiang, soy sauce, and mirin are made possible because of the nature of *A. oryzae* (and its closely related counterparts), but every one of them includes the hard work of microbes we're already very familiar with. *Aspergillus* is able to show off an impressive flexibility in range and flavor by facilitating yeast and bacteria, providing enzymes and nutrition they alone cannot, complementing their natural proclivities. In learning the nature of kōji, you will learn to wield all the microbes in this book at once.

KŌJI HISTORY

It is important to understand the traditions of kōji before getting creative with it. There is a long, intricate history with numerous varieties of *Aspergillus* weaving all over China, Japan, and Korea: *A. awamori*, *A. kawachii*, *A. kinzanji*, *A. usami*, *and A. sojae*, *Monascus* spp., *Mucor* spp., and *Rhizopus* spp., to name a few. The range and depth of this history and the traditions and cultures that come with them are astounding, and I highly recommend you spend time exploring more in the resources I've listed at the end of this book. The foundation of my knowledge on kōji comes from Japan, partly due to my own research and trials, and with special thanks to Haruko Uchishiba and her studies with the seven kōji producers of Japan. Therefore, the adaptations I've made for the following recipes are modeled on Japanese techniques and use some Japanese terminology.

A green-colored variety of *Aspergillus* called *kinzanji* (which is favored for protease production).

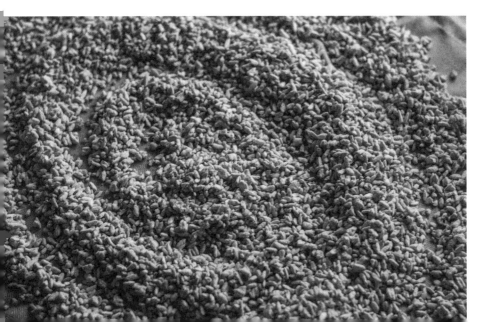

A block of rice knitted together with thick mycelial growth, collectively called kōji.

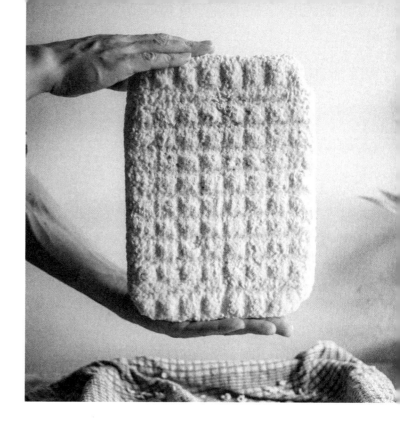

KŌJI

●
FERMENTER'S NOTE

As well as amylase and protease, Aspergillus *also produces lipase, an enzyme which is crucial to breaking down fats. In doing so, the trace amounts of fat in the substrates in this book will become fatty acids and not go rancid.*

Unlike the other forms of fermentation in this book, kōji moves between two basic stages: growth and application. The growth cycle lasts only 48 hours, which is a long time for a recipe but a very short time for fermentation. During this period, we have the opportunity to steer the direction of kōji, creating conditions that favor the production of very useful enzymes (amylase and protease), breaking down starch, protein, and fats into glucose, maltose, and amino acids (see Fermenter's Note, left). It is important to decide what you plan to make with the kōji in order to make sure the enzymes match your needs, or you can freestyle it and record the conditions that naturally occur, then decide the application accordingly. This rule also applies to the variety of *Aspergillus* you use, as they each have different strengths. Throughout the following recipes, I tend to use three varieties: *chohaku kairyo* (best suited for starch-based substrates, but is excellent for multiple types); *kinzanji* (for protein-rich substrates); and, of course, *oryzae* (superb for multiple substrates). I also use *Aspergillus kawachii* for amazake and shio kōji, where its citric acid production provides extra dimensions.

SOURCING SPORES

There are seven kōji spore producers in Japan, collectively supporting over 2,000 companies within the food and drink industry. The oldest was founded over 650 years ago, hailing from a time when there were hundreds of producers. Today, most of them are still family-owned, small-scale businesses. While it can be tricky to track down spores for international customers, there are an increasing number of producers outside of Japan that are happy to meet our demands. Be sure to check the variety of *Aspergillus* you're buying. Some aren't as well suited to particular ferments as others, while some are great for many uses.

GROWING KŌJI

The following steps apply to arborio rice, with notes on pearl barley adaptation. When dampening dish towels for use with kōji, pour freshly boiled water into a mixing bowl and carefully lower the towel in. Let it soak for a minute, then remove it and allow it to cool before wringing it out.

EQUIPMENT

steamer

steamer cloth

probe thermometer

powder shaker
  (optional)

insulated box

hot-water bottle or
  heating mat

INGREDIENTS

500g arborio rice

0.5g tane kōji
  (spores)

RICE PREPARATION

1. First, we wash and soak the rice for 24 hours. This is called *shinseki*, and it's a vital step in creating the right level of hydration within the grain and removes oxidized bran. Quickly wash the rice 8–10 times until the water is clear, then place in a bowl (large enough for the rice to expand as it soaks), cover with water 2in (5cm) above the rice, and leave it to soak at room temperature for 24 hours.

2. After 24 hours, drain and rinse the rice with fresh water, then leave it for 30 minutes–1 hour. At this stage, the rice should have gained 40–50 percent of its original weight and crumble when rubbed between your fingers.

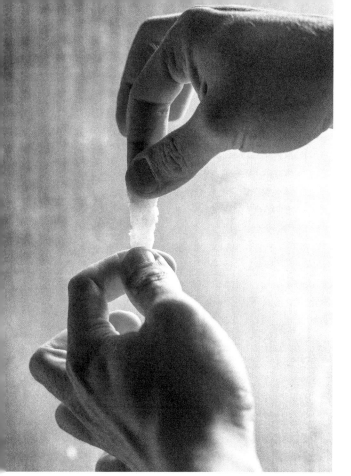

The stretch of perfectly steamed rice, called *gaiko-nainan*.

STEAMING

3. Line your steamer of choice with a steamer cloth (*kawashimaya*), or simply use a sieve set over a pan of boiling water. Once hot and steaming, add the rice layer by layer, one spoonful at a time. Wait for the rice to start turning opaque before adding the next layer, and continue until the steamer is full. This technique is called *nukegake* and allows for steam to flow evenly and freely between the grains.

4. Fold the cloth over the rice and cover with a lid. Mix the rice after 25 minutes to ensure even steaming, then cover and continue for another 25 minutes. The resulting texture of the rice is called *gaiko-nainan* (see right).

GAIKO-NAINAN

The term gaiko-nainan, *which describes the texture of the steamed rice, can only be described as a reverse* al dente. *If pasta should be soft on the outside with a firm texture within,* gaiko-nainan *describes rice that is firm on the outside and springy on the inside. This texture is one of the most important things to get right in preparing substrate for* kōji, *as the firm exterior provides a protective layer against pathogens. As previously mentioned, both bacteria and yeast can outspeed mold, but only mold can penetrate this style of firm steamed rice and access the nutrients within. To check if the rice is the perfect texture, squash a small amount into a ball as though you are making bread dough or mochi. The resulting ball should be stretchy like tight elastic. This rice ball is called* hinerimochi.

INOCULATION

5. *Tanekiri* is the name given to the application of spores to freshly steamed rice. Taking care not to burn yourself, pour the rice onto a clean, slightly damp dish towel and spread it out to cool off. To begin with, it is very hot, but it will quickly cool.

6. When it's about the temperature of a warm bath, inoculate with kōji spores. To do so evenly, use a powder shaker, a fine-mesh sieve, or even a tea infuser. Regular-sized sieve holes are far too big and will dump the spores all in one location. You need 1/1,000th the weight of your raw substrate in spores. To calculate this, multiply the weight of rice by 0.001. You can use up to three times this amount of spores if needed to cover all the rice, but don't exceed more than this or go lower.

7. The aim here is to be quick but also thorough. Spread the rice out in a thin layer and sprinkle the spores over the surface, working your way systematically over the whole area. Use a dough scraper to flip the rice over in sections and continue with the inoculation.

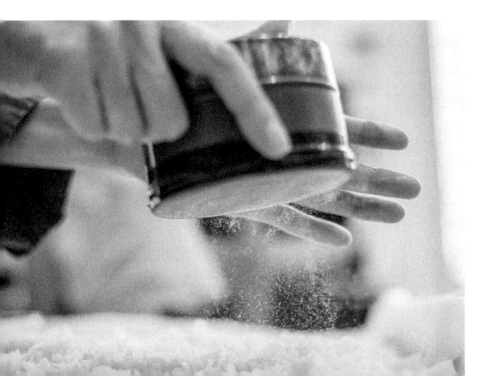

Steps 6–7, inoculating freshly steamed and cooled rice with kōji spores is a quick and thorough process. See Haruko in action in the photo.

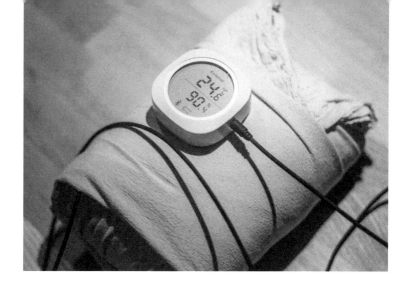

Step 9, the inoculated rice
is wrapped in two layers
with a temperature and
humidity probe, ready
for germination.

8. Repeat one more time until you've run out of spores.
   Now roll the mixture around with your hands to ensure
   a total and even distribution of spores over each grain
   of substrate. Take a note of the time—I usually start at
   10 A.M. and set alarms on my phone for the next stages.

GERMINATION

9. The most important factor for healthy germination of kōji
   is humidity. Pile the inoculated rice into a mound in the
   middle of the damp cloth and insert the thermometer.
   Tightly wrap the rice in the cloth, then follow up with a
   second cloth (here, I use a piece of canvas) to create a
   warm, moist environment. This is called *tsusumikomi*.

10. Place the wrapped-up rice in an insulated box (this can
    be the food box listed in the equipment section; see
    p.52) in a turned-off oven, or even a large lunch box
    wrapped in an electric blanket. At this stage, kōji must
    be kept around 86°F (30°C) and 90 percent humidity
    for 24 hours. Depending on the ambient temperature
    where you live, you may need to cool or heat the kōji.
    To cool it down, remove the lid of the box (or open the
    oven door); to warm it, store a hot-water bottle in the
    box with it, or use an electric heating mat from a home-
    brew supply store and lead the wires out under the lid.

11. Monitor the temperature of the kōji every couple of hours
    (while you're awake). You will only need to refresh the
    hot-water bottle once or twice during this initial 24 hours.

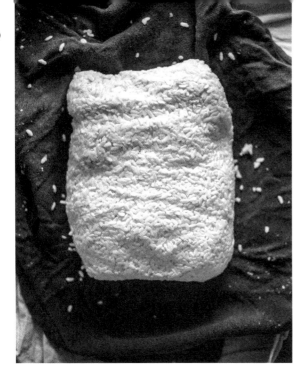

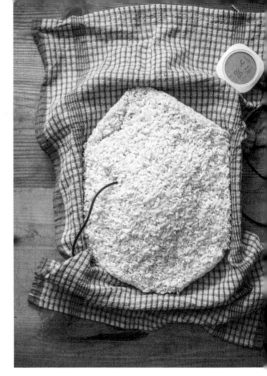

12 HOURS (86°F/30°C)

12. *Kirikaeshi* is an optional stage within the first 24-hour germination, which involves unwrapping the rice and breaking it up to control the rate of growth. You may find that, at this stage, the kōji temperature starts to climb by itself as it generates heat. Breaking up the rice will crash the temperature. You can then reshape the mound, insert the probe, and wrap it again for the remaining 12 hours.

24 HOURS (97°F/36°C)

13. The next stage, *mori*, is to mix and transfer the rice to a clean roasting pan with a clean rack in the bottom and a fresh dish towel beneath. This will allow air flow beneath the rice and keep condensed water away from directly making contact with it, where it can cause dampness. It's important that each grain of rice is rubbed free from neighboring grains, or they can soften and sour. At this stage, the rice will have white patches as the kōji grows and will have the sweet smell of chestnuts.

14. Shape the rice back into a mound in the roasting pan and reinsert the probe. Cover with another lightly dampened dish towel and place it back in the insulated box.

28 HOURS (100°F/38°C)

15. The next stage, *naka*, is to mix and spread the kōji out in the pan to form an even layer 1–1½in (3–4cm) thick (any thinner, and it will struggle to maintain temperature and moisture; too thick, and it will overheat internally), then return the probe beneath the rice and cover with a sheet of thick canvas or a clean, dry dish towel. This should be draped over the pan but not pressed in contact with the rice. By now, the rice should have about 50 percent coverage in white patches and will likely not need the assistance of a hot-water bottle. Return to the insulated box.

32 HOURS (104°F/40°C)

16. Mix the rice for a final time and spread it out again. This is called *shimai*.

17. Using your hands, create light furrows similar to a freshly plowed field running the length of the pan. Leave a few centimeters of unfurrowed rice at either end and reinsert the probe into the middle. This is the final mixing stage.

18. By now, the rice will have 80 percent coverage of kōji mold and be forming strong mycelial growth. The smell will also develop from a chestnut to more floral honeysuckle. The three mixing stages are collectively called *teire* and are good practice in growing kōji for an even and controlled enzyme production.

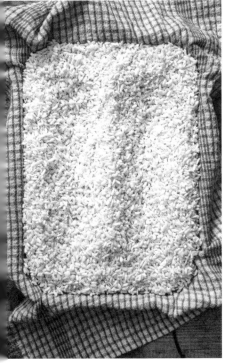
Step 17, *shimai*.

AMYLASE OR PROTEASE

These are the guideline temperatures and humidity for favorable amylase and protease production for Aspergillus oryzae. High levels of protease leads to savory and umami flavors and amylase leads to sweet, sugary flavors.

Amylase: 100–109°F (38–43°C) + 60–65 percent (low) humidity
Protease: 82–100°F (28–38°C) + 80–90 percent (high) humidity

Amylase production is actually broken down into two temperature ranges. The first is 100–104°F (38–40°C) for a-amylase, which produces a range of umami sweet flavors and causes liquefaction of starches. The second is 104–109°F (40–43°C) for gluco-amylase, which is purely sweet and produces glucose.
Kōji kept in conditions for amylase production will remain smoother and less fuzzy, while protease conditions produce a very thick mat. This is because the mold is driven to seek moisture within the grain, and the composition of grain tends to be protein on the outside and starch on the inside, leading kōji to produce the corresponding enzymes as required.

32–48 HOURS (LOADING ENZYMES)

19. During the final 15–16 hours, you have the option to create favorable conditions for amylase or protease production (see box, left). This is done by controlling the temperature and humidity of the kōji. Do this by adding the hot-water bottle to increase the temperature and placing a glass of water in the insulated box.

DRYING AND STORING

20. The process of stopping kōji at 48 hours, before it releases spores, is known as *dekōji*. Place a clean, dry piece of fabric over a table and spread the kōji out over it. Break up every grain by gently prying it apart and rolling it around on the fabric. It is traditionally laid out and marked with a spiral, leading from the middle.

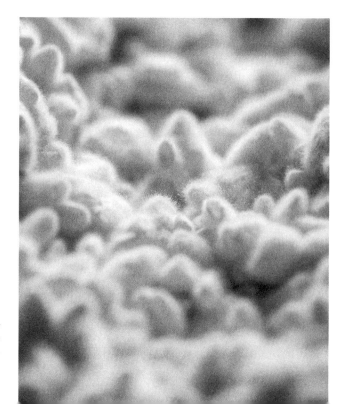

A macro shot of the fuzzy rice prior to breaking up the substrate for *dekōji*.

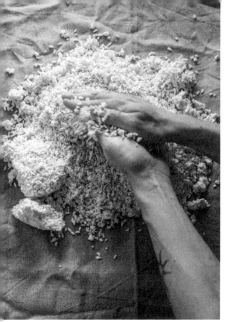

Step 20, break up every grain of rice to avoid trapped moisture during the drying process.

21. Leave it to cool and dry for a few hours, or use right away in your ferment of choice. At this stage, the kōji is loaded with enzymes and ready for use. Alternatively, you can pack the fresh kōji in an airtight container or vacuum bag and store it in the fridge for 2 weeks (or freeze for 3 months), or completely dry it out in a dehydrator. Once dried, it will keep for 1 year but be harder and tougher when mixing into smooth foods like miso.

SAVING SPORES

There are conflicting opinions over saving spores for future batches of kōji. While it is possible to do this, I am of the belief that it is more important to support the remaining producers of spores who do a lot of work to preserve pure lines of *Aspergillus*, as well as develop new lines. When saving spores at home, you risk the kōji changing over time, which can be hard to keep track of. But if this is something you're interested in, here's how to do it.

By following the previous steps, you can purposefully let kōji run to spore before drying it. If you ever find your kōji imparts a mushroomy flavor to your recipes, then chances are you've let it grow for too long and it's started sporing. This is why we break the kōji up at various intervals and closely control the moisture and temperature—to stop it from running to spore too quickly. In the hours following the 50-hour mark, kōji will spore, which you can then gently spread out and dry in the same method listed opposite. For this, I advise you wear latex gloves and a mask and make sure the room has no draft to disturb the spores. Let them dry out on the grain before vacuum sealing them or placing them in an airtight container with as little space for air as possible. Store them in a fridge for up to 2 weeks. To use them, add the grains into a powder shaker and apply as normal, knocking the spores loose as you shake. Dispose of the spent grain afterward.

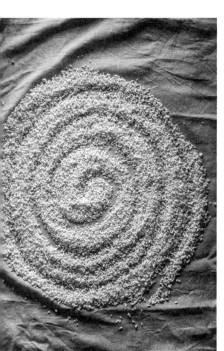

Step 20, *dekōji*. This is the traditional spiral shape made when drying kōji, which helps distribute moisture loss and temperature.

PEARL BARLEY AND ALTERNAT*IVE* RICES

If preparing pearl barley, the soaking time is 2–4 hours, depending on how well polished it is. Leave to drain for an hour before steaming, then steam for 30 minutes. The trick here is to make sure the barley isn't overhydrated. Unlike rice, barley has a tendency to absorb too much water, which can lead it to sour as lactic acid bacteria set in. When steamed, the barley should be springy and firm and not at all soft. Barley also comes in varying degrees of polish. I find that kōji struggles to grow in areas where more of the barley hull remains intact, so the more uniform and polished the barley, the better. Once steamed, follow the same steps for growing kōji (see p.166), but lower the overall temperature by 36°F (2°C) and spread out in a thin layer. Barley kōji is very oxygen-hungry and prone to overhumidification but also higher in protein than rice, so it's a great choice for amino acids and umami flavors.

You can use alternative rices, too, but make sure they're polished and you can easily wash the oxidized bran away. Steaming times will vary, but soak as normal for 24 hours, then leave to drain for an hour. When steaming, check on the rice every 20 minutes and mix it to create a uniform finish. Rices like bomba have great moisture retention, but long grain has improved airflow. Don't be afraid to experiment and have fun.

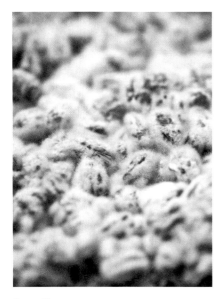

Aspergillus grown on pearl barley.

APPLICATION

Once armed with kōji, a whole world of applications opens up to you. In its dried stage, kōji substrate (rice and barley) can be infused in oils, simmered in stock, and ground into a flour and used to *pané* all manner of fried foods. Outside of the more conventional recipes, the world is your oyster. Add a handful of fully grown rice kōji at the start of any of the lacto ferment recipes in this book and experience how the enzymes unlock more flavor than you imagined possible. You can even roast it like coffee. So go wild.

KŌJI ENZYMES

Enzymes also have their optimum temperatures when applied to different recipes:

Amylase: 131–140°F (55–60°C)
Protease: 86–104°F (30–40°C)

Amylase applications tend to be fast acting, while protease can take a lot longer. For example, the miso recipes in this book (see p.191) are ready at the earliest in 6 months, and the shoyu (see p.202) takes even longer. The amazake (see p.176) is ready in 12 hours. These temperatures are a guide for optimum conditions, but the recipes will work in suboptimal conditions, as long as it isn't so hot the enzymes denature. Temperature is more important during the first 48 hours of kōji-making than later on.

   Another point of interest in the application of kōji is your choice of substrate. The level of starch versus protein will affect the resulting flavor through the creation of natural sweetness and umami respectively, so swapping out soybean for split pea will make a world of difference, even within the same recipe and conditions—see table below.

INGREDIENT (RAW)	PROTEIN (PER 100G)	CARBOHYDRATE (PER 100G)
Soybean	40g	30g
Fava bean	8g	18g
Lima bean	8g	21g
Pinto/navy bean	21g	63g
Kidney bean	24g	60g
Cannellini bean	23g	60g
Black bean	8.8g	24g
Chickpea	19g	61g
Split pea	25g	60g
Lentil	9g	20g
Rice	2.4g	29g
Barley	12g	73g
Wheat (durum)	14g	71g
Spelt	15g	70g
Rye	9.8g	77g
Oat	13g	67g

AMAZAKE

EQUIPMENT

yogurt machine,
    rice cooker,
    multicooker, or
    sous-vide machine

SWEET AMAZAKE

300g cooked rice

100g rice kōji

100g water

STRONG AMAZAKE

300g rice kōji

150g water

The fastest kōji ferment, amazake offers a huge range in flavor, applications, and additional options to truly make it your own. Sweet in a wonderfully complex way, amazake really demonstrates the power of enzymes. When we think of sweet, sugar comes to mind, but sugar is a flat, one-dimensional sweetness. Amazake offers nuance and breadth in sweetness due to how the enzyme "cuts" up the starch. Unlike a lot of sweet flavors made from uniform molecules, amazake has a randomizing nature, breaking some molecules down into shorter forms and others longer. We taste each and every one of these. Strong amazake has a powerful kōji flavor, which can take over other ingredients.

For the rice kōji, you can try *A. chohaku*, *A. oryzae*, or *A. kawachii* (along with any amylase-specializing variety) to experience completely different results. Once made, amazake is traditionally consumed as a sweet drink served hot or cold, or it can be added into dressings, breakfasts, or smoothies. You can also add 1–2 percent salt to turn amazake into a savory marinade, somewhat akin to shio kōji (see p.182), but less salty.

FERMENTER'S NOTE

When adding amazake to other recipes, note that the enzymes may have unexpected effects on other foods. For example, it will liquidize starchy ingredients like potatoes and rice, dissolve gluten in flour-based foods, and stop gelatin from setting.

1. Mix the ingredients together and add them to a yogurt machine, rice cooker, or multicooker, or you can use a sous-vide machine. Set to "keep warm," or 86–131°F (30–55°C)—it must stay below 135°F (57°C)—for 12 hours, stirring once or twice during the process.

2. After 12 hours, the amazake will have broken down the rice and become far smoother. You can eat it as is, blend it until completely smooth, or pass it through a sieve to remove any remaining solid grains. It is now ready to use, or it can be stored chilled in the fridge for 1–2 months.

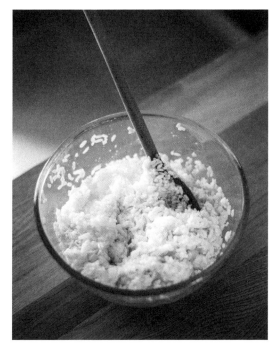

Step 1.

AMAZAKE ICE CREAM

Mix 2–3 tablespoons of smooth amazake into 200ml of cream before churning your favorite ice cream recipe.

AMAZAKE FRENCH TOAST

Mix 100g amazake and milk in equal parts with a pinch of cinnamon and an egg. Whisk, then soak sliced bread in it for 10 minutes before frying in a hot pan with butter.

AMAZAKE YOGURT

Add a few tablespoons to your homemade yogurt (see p.105) and use to top a fruit salad.

AMAZAKE SMOOTHIE

Stir a few tablespoons into your favorite smoothie for a flavor boost.

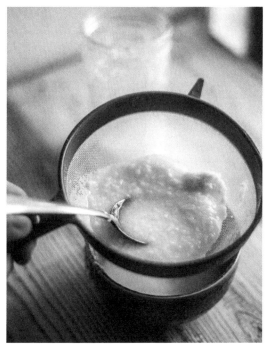

Step 2, passing through a sieve.

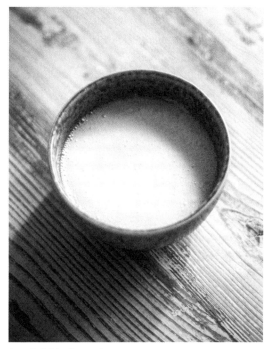

Step 2, finished amazake.

AMAZAKE VARIATIONS

Why not try replacing the cooked rice with cooked oats or rye? Tailor your amazake to the grains locally available to you and see how it tastes.

There is plenty of scope for creativity with amazake, whether savory or sweet, from swapping out the water for fruit juices, vegetable purées, milk, or nut milk to infusing the water with teas or including spices and herbs.

You can enjoy amazake as a hot or cold drink as it is or add it into the kombucha cream recipe (see p.142) instead of sugar or honey. I designed the following recipes to serve two and used sweet amazake (not strong).

INGREDIENTS

500ml whole milk
(or milk alternative)

250g sweet amazake
(see p.176)

2 tbsp light tahini

juice of 1 lemon

½ tsp vanilla paste

pinch of salt (optional)

grated lemon zest and
honey, to serve

SESAME AND LEMON AMAZAKE

Nutty, sweet, and refreshing. Try different types of citrus for alternative flavors, and mix fresh rose petals in for additional fragrance. These go particularly well with bergamot lemon.

Place all the ingredients apart from the zest and honey in a blender and blend until smooth. Pour into an airtight container and store in the fridge overnight (or a minimum of 2 hours). Divide between two cups, top with the lemon zest, and sweeten with honey to taste. Serve chilled.

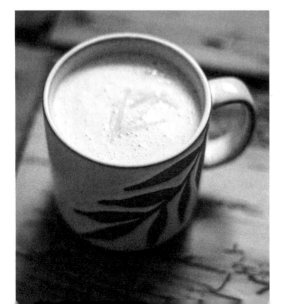

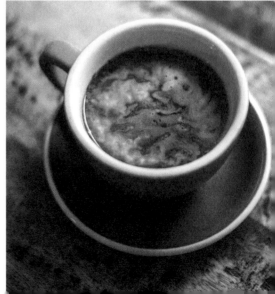

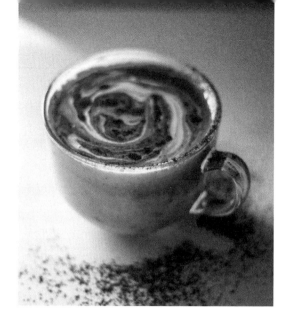

Left Raspberry amazake.

p.178 left Sesame and lemon amazake.

p.178 right Coffee amazake.

INGREDIENTS

500ml milk

80g yogurt (see p.105 or use natural yogurt)

250g sweet amazake (see p.176)

200g raspberries

pinch of salt (omit if using lacto berry powder)

lacto berry powder (optional, see p.83)

RASPBERRY AMAZAKE

This recipe works with any seasonal berry or currants, fresh or frozen. Make a thicker version and enjoy it as a topping to your breakfast with toasted hazelnuts. If you've made lacto berry powder, use it to dust the top.

Blend all the ingredients except for the berry powder. Once smooth, chill in a fridge overnight (or a minimum of 2 hours). Divide between two cups and serve dusted with lacto berry powder over the surface.

INGREDIENTS

200ml milk

160g sweet amazake (see p.176)

60g espresso

dark chocolate (optional)

COFFEE AMAZAKE

I like my coffee black, but even I have to admit that amazake and coffee are a match made in heaven. Think affogato meets cortado. And for the chocolate lovers, add a pinch of cocoa powder, or better yet, melt a block of dark chocolate into your espresso before adding it to the amazake.

To serve chilled, blend the milk and amazake together and place in a fridge for 2 hours. Divide between two cups and pour the espresso over the top.

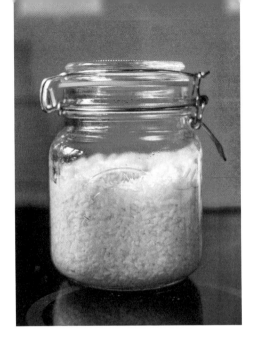
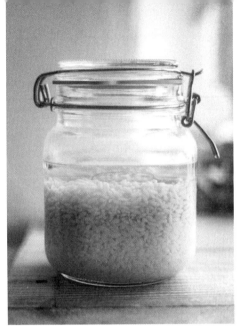

Freshly made mirin looks dry (left), but as the enzymes break down the rice, more liquid is released, sweetening the alcohol (right).

MIRIN

EQUIPMENT

2-liter jar with an airtight lid

glass or ceramic weight

2 × 1-liter bottles

ADAPTED MEASUREMENTS:

580g cooked and cooled glutinous rice

700ml vodka

120g rice kōji (see p.166)

TRADITIONAL MEASUREMENTS:

580g cooked and cooled glutinous rice

330ml shochu or vodka

65g rice kōji (see p.166)

Comparable to a sweet cooking wine, mirin is high in natural sugars, so it comes into its own when used to make sauces, marinades, and stocks—and it is ideal for glazes. I'm going to make a bold statement and say, unless you are very lucky or determined, chances are you've never tasted traditional mirin. This is because of the wide selection of mirinlike products and seasonings available that can be tricky to discern between. This was due to postwar restrictions and prohibition of alcohol production in Japan. Traditional mirin is at once very simple to make, but takes a long time to age. It was originally made with shochu, a Japanese distilled beverage with an alcohol content of 25 percent. This recipe recreates the original by using vodka, more commonly available in this part of the world, and scales down measurements for ease of home production. If you can get your hands on shochu, then more power to you; the following recipe will work perfectly either way.

1. Put the cooled, cooked glutinous rice into a mixing bowl. Add the vodka and rice kōji, and mix.

2. Pour all of it into the jar and carefully add a weight. It doesn't need to be heavy, but enough to hold the rice down. Secure with an airtight lid and leave the jar somewhere out of the way at room temperature for 3 months (adapted measurements) or 6 months (traditional measurements).

3. Filter the liquid (mirin) from the rice. Transfer the mirin to bottles and continue to age for at least another 3 months (or up to 9 months more, bringing it to a full year) for adapted measurements and for another 12 months for traditional measurements. During this period, it will darken and mature as it ages. It will keep for years—and just gets better and better.

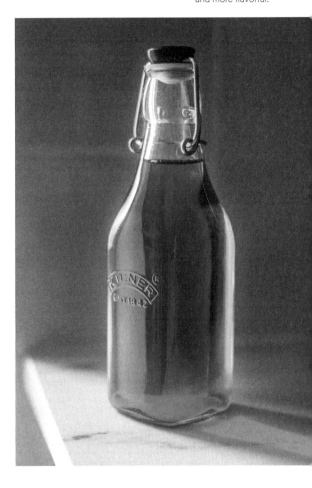

Once bottled, mirin will continue to age and grow gradually darker and more flavorful.

MIRIN VARIATIONS

For additional flavors, infuse the vodka with fruit or berries before using it to make mirin. Because vodka has a higher percentage of alcohol, it is safe to infuse with 200g of fruit in the adapted recipe (but not in the traditional recipe, as it's very dry and the liquid from the fruit could dilute the alcohol enough to spoil it).

You can also use other spirits, such as whisky, for delicious and interesting drinks, as well as fantastic cooking mirin.

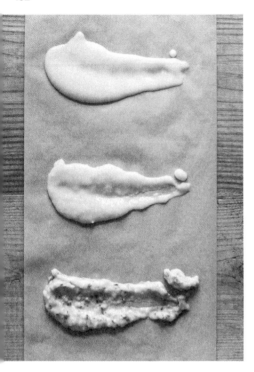

Plain shio kōji (top), lemon zest shio kōji (middle), and shiitake shio kōji (bottom); each offering a unique opportunity to imbue other ingredients with powerful flavors.

SHIO KŌJI

Many of us know to salt meat or vegetables ahead of cooking. The act breaks down cells and draws out moisture while seasoning an ingredient from within. Now imagine supercharging this process by loading it with kōji enzymes; I give you shio kōji (meaning "salt kōji"). Considered a condiment, shio kōji has a vast number of applications in the kitchen, from seasoning to marinating or pickling. It can also be mixed with other ingredients to meld flavors together precooking. While it might seem like there is a lot of salt used here, it is important for the function and safety of shio kōji. It is also worth remembering that a recipe will never call for much. So if shio kōji is 10 percent salt and a recipe only called for 10g shio kōji, then you're only using 1g salt.

EQUIPMENT

1-liter jar with an airtight lid

INGREDIENTS

500g rice kōji

100g sea salt (10%)

500g water

1. Rub the kōji and salt together and pour them into the jar. Fill with water and mix well.

2. Fasten an airtight lid in place and continue to stir daily until the rice is roughly broken down. This will take about 2 days.

3. Store in the fridge for later use. Alternatively, you can use an immersion blender to create a smooth, uniform shio kōji or pass it through a sieve, if you want to avoid lumps. It will keep in the fridge for up to 4 months.

SHIO KŌJI VARIATIONS

There are many versions of shio kōji you can make, each offering powerful culinary applications. From a super-charged, heavily fragrant version to versions infused with mushroom umami, citrus, alliums, or herbs, each one is packed with flavor and those all-important enzymes.

SWEET AND UMAMI SHIO KŌJI

Follow steps 1–2 (opposite), then keep the shio kōji warm (at 104–122°F/40–50°C) for 6 hours. You can do this in a multicooker set to "ferment" or in the insulated box used to grow kōji, or place the container of shio kōji in a dehydrator set to 104°F (40°C), but keep its lid on to keep it from getting dried out. After 6 hours, mix and store in a fridge.

FLAVORED SHIO KŌJI

Mix the rice kōji, salt, and flavoring ingredient together in a bowl, then add the water and stir, and proceed to follow steps 2–3 of shio kōji (opposite). To use the flavored shio kōji, I weigh the prepared ingredients I want to cure and calculate 10–15 percent of that weight. (For example, for 200g meat, I would use 20–30g flavored shio kōji. Generally speaking, 10 percent is used for vegetables and 15 percent for meat or fish.) I then apply this much shio kōji to the prepared ingredients and leave at room temperature for an hour before cooking. When cooking, take care, as foods will burn more easily.

INGREDIENTS

200g rice kōji

50g sea salt (10%)

100g flavoring ingredient (such as garlic, onion, mushroom, citrus, ginger root, or fresh herbs, finely chopped, crushed, or blended as applicable)

200g water

COOKING WITH FERMENTS

PICKLING WITH SHIO KŌJI

Clean and roughly chop your choice of vegetables, tofu, boiled egg, or mushroom; add 15 percent shio kōji; mix well; cover and store it in an airtight container for 1 hour–1 day.

SHIO KŌJI IN SAUCES AND JAMS

Add 10 percent shio kōji to sauces, such as tomato, BBQ, sriracha, or mole instead of seasoning with salt to unlock more flavor with enzymes. The shio kōji can be cooked into the sauce or added at the end (once cooled), which will preserve its enzymes and unlock more flavor over time. It will, however, shorten the shelf life of the sauce to 3 months, depending on the sauce, and require refrigeration. Adding 3 percent to homemade jams is also amazing.

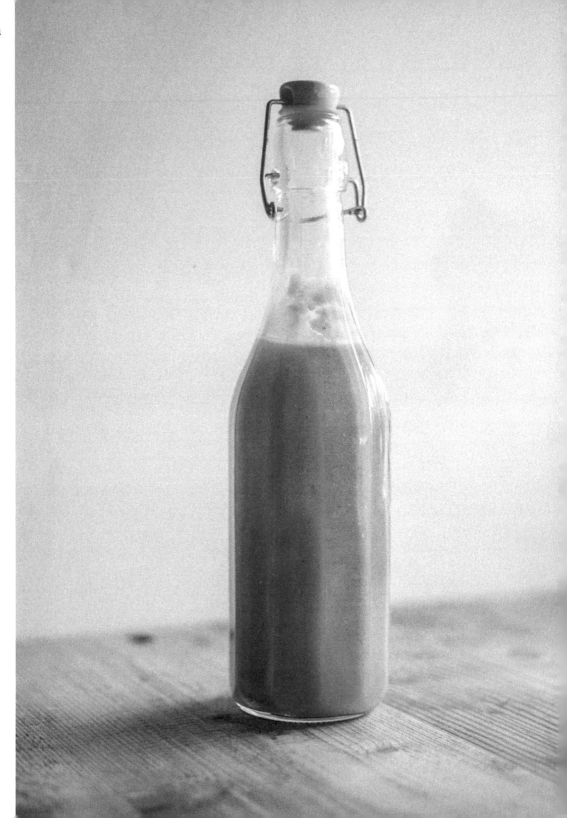

KŌJI HOT SAUCE

EQUIPMENT

1-liter jar with an airtight lid

weight

INGREDIENTS

1kg tomatoes (see
  Fermenter's Note)

2 garlic cloves, sliced

7 chilies, halved
  lengthwise

2in (5cm) ginger root,
  sliced

100g kōji (see p.166)

smoked salt (3%)

FERMENTER'S NOTE

*Swap out some of the tomato
for other ingredients to make
this hot sauce your own, but
if you're working with drier
ingredients, remember to add
enough water to cover them
and include it when calculating
the amount of salt to add. It
also works especially well
with mixtures of fruits such
as mango, charred pineapple,
and peaches.*

There are a million and one hot sauce recipes out there, and the beauty of fermented hot sauce is the balancing action of acidity on spice. As the lactic acid bacteria (LAB, see p.64) does its job (sometimes with a little help from *Brettanomyces*, depending on how many tomatoes you've added, see p.68), the lactic acid balances the spice, allowing you to use higher quantities and enjoy the flavor without blowing your head off. It also nicely demonstrates the "chuck some kōji in, too" technique, which flushes the ingredients with kōji enzymes, unlocking more flavor and complexity than you'd get from a regular lacto-fermented hot sauce.

1. Clean, weigh, and prepare all the ingredients and mix in the smoked salt. This recipe will work with regular salt, but I love the addition of smokiness. Place them in the clean jar and apply a weight to compress them.

2. Secure an airtight lid and leave it at room temperature for 2 days, then begin burping the jar (see p.67), as gas will likely build up significantly in the initial stages.

3. Continue burping the jar for another 5 days (1 week in total), when the pH should have reached 3.5.

4. Move the hot sauce to a fridge to slow down the activity and let it age for another week.

5. Blend until smooth, then bottle and store it in the fridge. Use it within 3 months, or freeze for up to 1 year.

Step 3, kōji hot sauce prior to aging in the fridge.

A dark and delicious porcini garum, which is made from porcini gifted to me by a forager friend, Aimée.

Originally from ancient Rome (garum) and ancient Greece (garos), garum is traditionally a fermented fish sauce, where fish (along with its blood and guts) and salt are packed into a vessel and left out in the sun. The fish's own digestive enzymes decompose it in an act of self-digestion called autolysis, which, given enough time, produces a complex and umami sauce similar to modern-day fish sauce or soy sauce. And yes, the smell was so potent that laws were passed in ancient Rome banning the production of garum in close proximity to towns and settlements.

For this recipe, we'll make a version using mushrooms. By applying the enzymes of kōji to mushrooms, we can somewhat recreate this act of digestion, fungus on fungus. While this isn't strictly a garum, it also isn't strictly a fish sauce, soy sauce, or shoyu either. Instead, it occupies a space between these and a lactic acid bacteria ferment, which nicely speeds it up so you only have to wait 4–5 weeks.

PORCINI GARUM

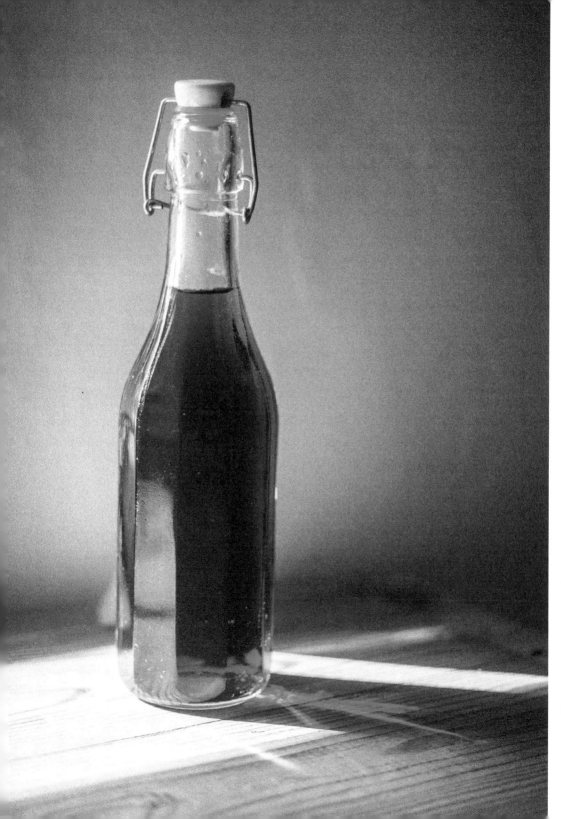

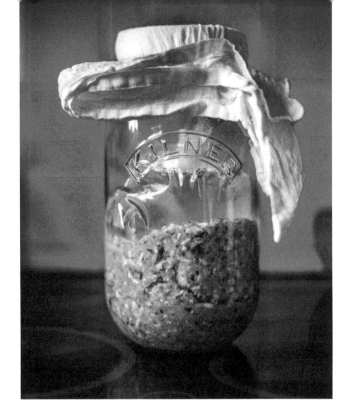

Step 2, prior to fermentation.

● FERMENTER'S NOTE

The porcini mushrooms in this recipe can be dried or fresh. If using dried, fully hydrate them in cold water and use this water as part of the water in the recipe. Inoculate the ferment with ginger root, garlic, or whey to introduce lactic acid bacteria. You can also use any edible mushrooms—shiitake are good— and substitute up to 10 percent of the mushrooms for aromatic ingredients like herbs, garlic, onion, or ginger.

EQUIPMENT

2.5-liter jar

fabric lid

string or elastic band

food-safe plastic bag

INGREDIENTS

320g kōji (see p.166)

132g salt (5.5%)

480g water

1.6kg porcini mushrooms
(see Fermenter's Note)

1. Begin by pulsing the kōji, salt, and water together in a blender until the rice is broken up. Add the mushrooms and continue to pulse until they're broken up but not a smooth paste.

2. Transfer the mixture to the large sanitized jar, then fill the plastic bag with either spare grain or water and seal it. Squeeze the bag on top of the garum to hold the pulp down below the surface of the liquid and secure the fabric over the mouth of the jar.

3. Leave it at 68–77°F (20–25°C) for at least 4–5 weeks, opening to the jar and stirring once a week. If cooler, ferment for longer. After the first few weeks, give it a sniff. If all goes well, it should smell of a deep, nutty umami, similar to cooked mushrooms.

4. After 5 weeks have passed, you can either filter out the solids and bottle the garum liquid or move the whole jar somewhere cooler and continue to age. There is a balancing act with this ferment, where the kōji will continue to unlock flavor, but the LAB will make it more sour. The final results can range anywhere from a light mushroomy soy sauce to a deeply umami kraut brine.

5. Once made, store in a fridge for up to 4 months and use like you would soy sauce. Boiling or frying with it will destroy the delicate aroma, but frying will unlock extra levels of deep umami. Take care not to burn it, though. For long-term storage, seal it in a freezer-safe container and freeze.

Step 4, ready to filter out the solids.

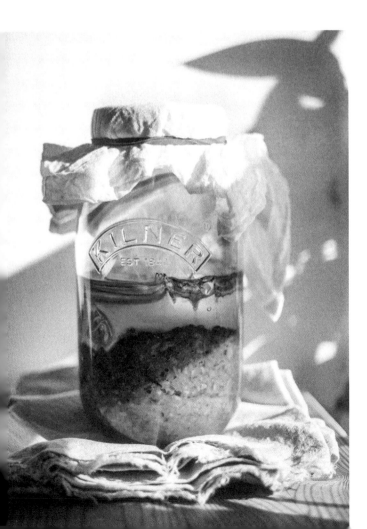

ICE CLARIFICATION

Ice clarification is a process of extracting an incredibly clear liquid from the pulp of fermentation. Doing so preserves the best flavor, as sediment often releases bitterness when heated. I'd reserve ice clarification for ferments that are completely finished, as freezing live microbes will dampen their mood and likely halt any further fermentation. It works well for garums and shoyu. Pour the ferment into a freezer-safe box and freeze until solid, then secure a piece of muslin or a dish towel over a bowl and place the frozen block on top of it. Cover with a lid to avoid contamination from pests or debris and let thaw at room temperature. As the ice melts, it drips through the fabric, leaving behind the solid matter and producing a remarkable clear liquid. Bottle the liquid and treat as the original recipe suggests.

COOKING
WITH FERMENTS

PORCINI GARUM GLAZE

Brush it onto rice or onto whitefish, such as halibut, flounder, or sole.

SCRAMBLED EGGS

There are a million and one ways people love their eggs, but you have to try a few drops of mushroom garum on scrambled eggs or inside an omelet before folding it.

TO DEGLAZE A PAN

When sautéing fresh vegetables or making fried rice, splash a little mushroom garum in the pan toward the end of cooking to lift any sticky residue back off the pan and into the sauce.

SAUCES OR STOCK

Add to cream sauces or stock for an extra boost.

MARINADE

Use to marinate vegetables and animal protein, infusing them with a delicate mushroomy flavor.

GARUM
VARIATIONS

These all work with the same measurements as the recipe on p.186. Simply swap out the fresh mushroom for the equal weight in the ingredients listed below:
- Tomato and seaweed
- Rye bread or old sourdough
- Onion peel and peppercorn

You can also make alternative mushroom garums by using a mixture of mushroom varieties or swapping out 100g of mushrooms for an aromatic plant, such as wild garlic, chili pepper, or celery.

MISO (AMINO PASTE)

One of the kings of umami and one of the few examples of solid-state fermentation in this book, miso comes in many deeply savory forms. Within the world of traditional miso, there is the sweet, pale shiro; the fruity and rich mugi; and almost black hatcho (to name just a few).

In the last decade, miso has been unleashed upon the world in extraordinary fashion, with experimental adaptations of the technique being applied to local crops across the globe. The main criteria for making miso is protein, but when made from a nontraditional substrate (usually soybeans, rice, and barley), we tend to use the name "amino paste," in reference to the coveted amino acids produced during fermentation. There have also been a host of playful names invented for new staple amino pastes, largely thanks to NOMA, who I credit with the invention of "peaso" and "breadso," miso made using split peas and bread.

Amino pastes can be made with a whole range of beans, peas, grains, and seeds, thanks to their high levels of protein. See the chart in the section on kōji application (p.175) for a full breakdown. We grow a lot of fava beans in the garden, which are then dried. These make excellent miso, as do lima beans (making a quicker, sweet miso), and, of course, soybeans. There are multiple styles of miso, which adjust the ratio of rice kōji to cooked bean, as well as versions (hatcho) that require the growth of *Aspergillus* on the soybeans themselves. The following recipe works for soybeans, lima beans, fava beans, yellow split peas, and chickpeas. For legumes with lower protein content (see p.175), replace the rice kōji with barley kōji, as the additional protein from the barley will help boost the umami in the final miso.

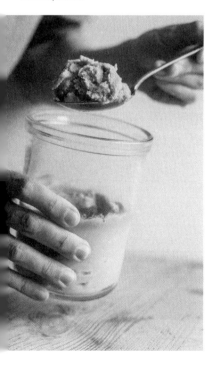

A smooth, 6–7-month-aged white miso, made from soybeans.

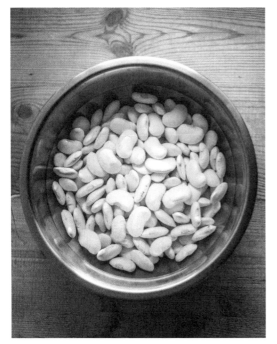

Step 1.

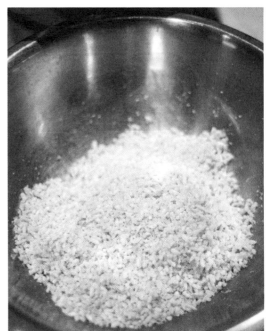

Step 4.

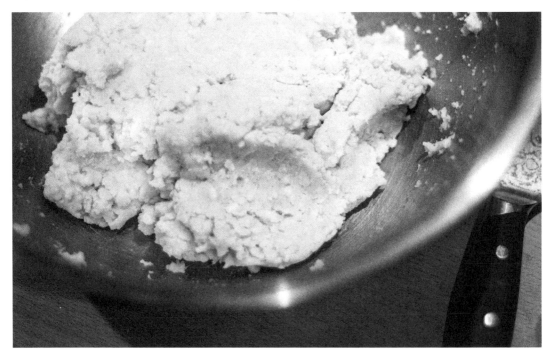

Step 5.

1-liter jar or crock with
  a lid

INGREDIENTS

270g dried beans

500g kōji (rice or barley,
  see p.166)

100g sea salt (10–15%)

1 tbsp wasabi paste

1. Begin by preparing the beans. To do so, pick through them, removing damaged or soft beans, then soak them in twice their volume of water for 3–6 hours.

2. Drain and let them dry for 1–2 hours, then boil gently for 35–40 minutes (or longer, depending on the variety you use—if making traditional miso with soybeans, cook for 5–6 hours). Do not let them rapidly boil as you want to cook them throughout without overcooking the outside. Much like most kōji ferments, moisture is very important. The beans are done when they can be crushed between the thumb and pinky finger to produce a fluffy starch. To test this with accuracy, place one bean on some scales. Press it gently with one finger and see how much pressure is required to pop it open. The scales should not exceed 500g, and ideally (depending on the variety of bean) require 300–450g pressure. If the bean is too tough or the starch feels chalky, then continue to cook for another 5–10 minutes. Avoid overcooking, as this will introduce too much water and cause your miso to sour or turn alcoholic.

3. Drain the cooked beans and then use a fork, potato masher, large pestle and mortar, meat grinder, or food processor to coarsely grind them. Reserve some of the liquid from the cooked beans to add back into the paste if it becomes too dry when crushing. You're looking to make a paste that is moist enough to form into balls but not so damp that liquid comes back out when pressed. (As a rough guide, most fully hydrated beans should have increased in weight by 50–60 percent from dried.)

4. Add the fresh rice kōji and salt to a separate bowl and rub them together to break up the rice and disperse the salt.

5. Pour the kōji and salt mixture into the bean paste and continue to mash for 5 minutes until everything is thoroughly combined. (Note that some beans have a tougher skin than others. If you find it impossible to grind them, continue with the next stage anyway. Once the miso is a few months old, you can unpack it, remash, and repack it again, as the enzymes will have softened everything.) In total, the amount of kōji to bean can be 70–100 percent by weight, so you have wiggle room if you have cooked too many beans.

6. Roll the mash into balls (about 200g) and test if they're the right hydration by throwing one against the inside of the bowl. If correct, the ball will impact and stick without cracking (see image).

7. Now press each ball firmly, one by one, into the clean glass jar or crock. Layer them up, working from the bottom, making sure to compress them so that no air or cracks are visible. Any gaps are vulnerable to unwanted mold growth.

8. Once all the mash is in place, smooth the top off and cover the surface with a piece of parchment paper, pressing it tightly to the miso to block out oxygen. Put the wasabi paste on top of the parchment paper, cover the mouth of the jar with plastic wrap, and remove the rubber seal from the lid. Secure the lid over the plastic wrap. By removing the seal, we allow air pressure inside to escape but trap the wasabi vapor within.

9. Place the container somewhere warm (68–77°F/ 20–25°C) for the fastest results, but it can be left at any ambient temperature.

●

THE WASABI METHOD

This wasabi method was shown to me by Haruko. The combination of the salt already inside the miso and a volatile compound given off by the wasabi, allyl isothiocyanate, proves to be a truly hostile environment to unwelcome microbes. Allyl isothiocyanate fills the remaining air between the surface of the miso and the layer of plastic wrap while still allowing the container to breathe when gas needs to escape. It's important not to let carbon dioxide build in the vessel, as this can impart unpleasant flavors in the miso.

●

FERMENTER'S NOTE

If you don't have wasabi, you can sprinkle a pinch of extra salt over the surface, add a piece of parchment paper or plastic wrap over the surface, then apply a weight on top that's roughly equal to half the weight of the miso itself. Add a lid that can be a breathable cloth or a lid with no rubber seal. This technique will still allow the surface to grow mold, which should be scraped away before eating.

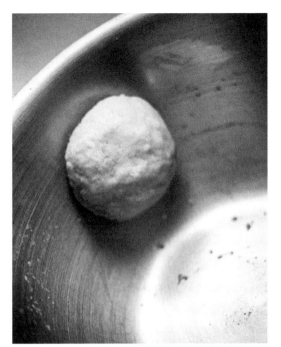

Step 6.

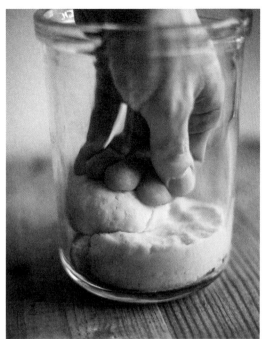

Step 7.

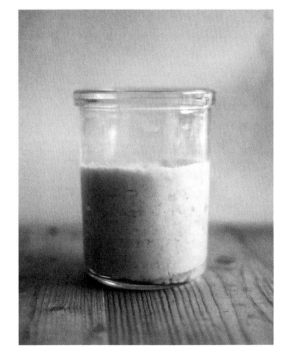

Step 8, smoothed surface.

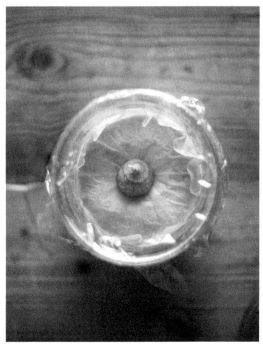

Step 8, covered surface.

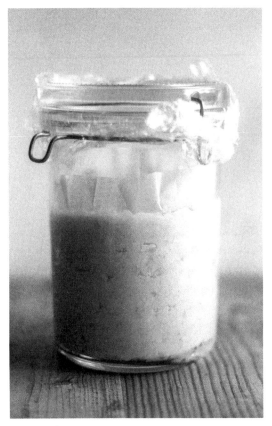

Freshly made miso.

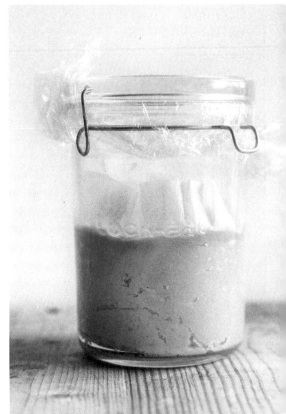

6-month-old miso.

10. After the first week, a reddish-pink liquid may appear on top of the miso. This is tamari, a sauce you may already be familiar with. (It can be used like soy sauce or shoyu.)

11. After 2–3 weeks, the miso should smell almost buttery and fruity with a salty umami.

12. Continue to ferment for at least 6 months before tasting. Don't worry if mold grows on the surface. Simply scrape back the top layer when the miso is ready to eat, or, if it appears early in the ferment, remove and discard the mold and repack the miso in a clean jar.

13. Once ready, store it in the fridge to slow down further development of flavor. Store in an airtight container in a fridge, where it will last 1 year.

COOKING WITH FERMENTS

MISO SOUP

Stir in a spoonful of miso to a brothy soup once the pan is removed from the heat.

MISO PICKLED VEGETABLES

Coat cleaned raw vegetables in a small amount of miso and leave them to pickle for 2–3 hours for a lightly seasoned, fruity side dish.

MISO MASH

Swap out salt or cheese for miso when mashing potatoes with butter. Thank me later.

MISO CARAMEL

Make your favorite caramel recipe, but after adding the cream, add 1–2 tbsp of white miso and whisk. Forget salted caramel. Note you can do the same when making fudge.

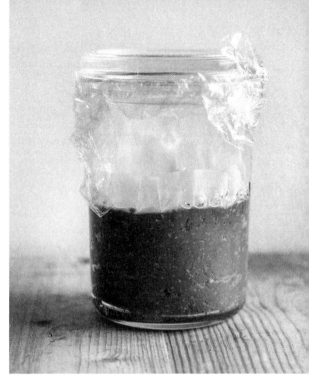

My homemade version of mugi miso.

MISO VARIATIONS

Miso comes in a few different varieties. Here are some alternatives for the rice kōji when making miso.

HATCHO MISO

An alternative version of miso is called hatcho miso, and it's deeply umami with rich balsamic notes. The key difference here is that the soybeans are used as a substrate to grow the kōji after adding salt and mashing into a paste, often with toasted spelt or wheat flour. Hatcho is also often much dryer, saltier, and aged for 3 years.

MUGI MISO

This type of miso is made with barley kōji. Decrease the amount of kōji to 35:65 ratio with cooked soybeans. This type of miso is a pungent, deep-red miso thanks to the additional barley protein, aged for longer (10 months), and suits both winter and summer recipes.

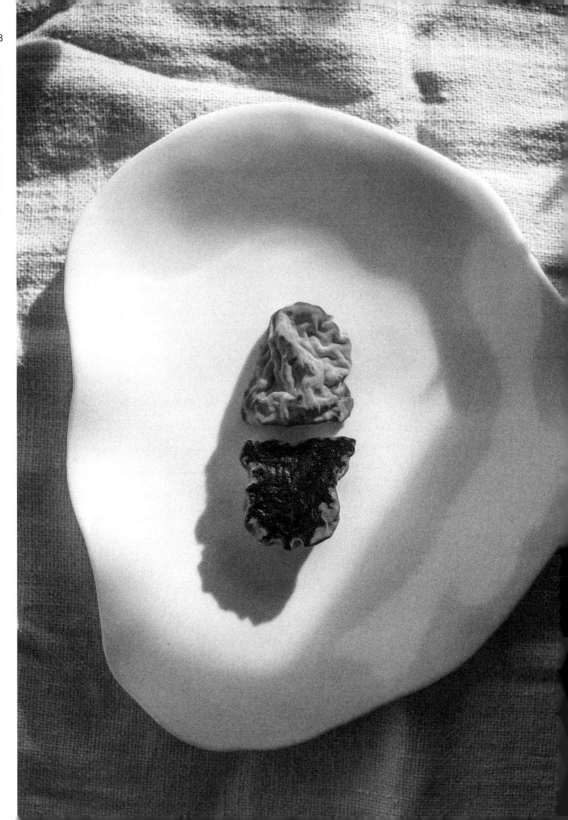

Kōji-cured beet
charcuterie holds as
much flavor as you
can pack into it.

_____

EQUIPMENT

vacuum sealer

powder shaker

insulated box

probe thermometer

hot-water bottle or heat mat

dehydrator

smoker (optional)

INGREDIENTS

4 large beets

½ tsp mixed cracked
   peppercorns

10ml balsamic vinegar

smoked salt (2%; see
   Fermenter's Note, p.201)

kōji spores (see p.166)

Rich and umami in flavor and with a wonderful texture, kōji-cured vegetables offer an alternative to cured meats that are much quicker to produce and versatile in flavor. All root vegetables that I've tried have worked, although some are tastier than others. I chose beets, here, for their sweetness, texture, and color. The key to this technique is moisture. If a vegetable is too wet, bacteria like LAB will run wild; if it's too dry, the kōji won't have enough moisture to get going.

This is probably one of the most advanced recipes in this book and requires most of the equipment listed in Getting Set Up (see pp.42–55). Once made, these last for a month. They make an amazing showstopper for plant-based charcuterie and a delicious addition to broths, salads, and all things between two slices of bread.

KŌJI
CHARCUTERIE
VEGETABLES

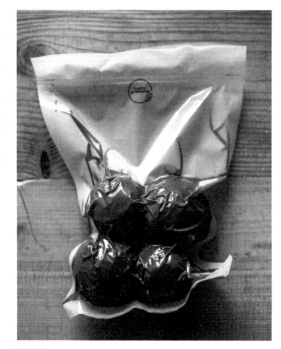

Step 2.

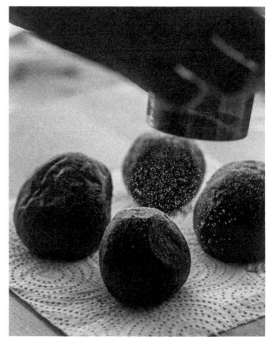

Step 4, inoculating the beets with kōji.

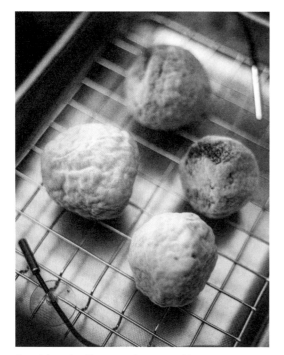

Step 4, inoculated beets starting to turn white.

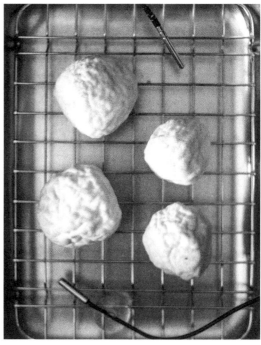

Step 4, inoculated beets after 48 hours.

1. First off, boil the beets until cooked through, then smoke them for 10–20 minutes to infuse with more flavor. Alternatively, you can slow roast them whole (skin on) at 400°F (200°C) for 45–60 minutes.

2. Peel the beets, then vacuum seal them with the peppercorns, vinegar, and salt. Leave them to cure in a fridge for 3–5 days.

3. Remove the beets from the vacuum packaging and pat them dry.

4. Inoculate with kōji spores using the powder shaker to make sure they have an even distribution, then place them on a wire rack in the insulated box. Using a probe and hot-water bottle (or heat mat), maintain a temperature of 82–91°F (28–33°C) for the full 48-hour growth cycle of kōji. During this time, the kōji will produce its characteristic fuzz all over the beets, taking on its pink hue before turning white.

5. Once done, dehydrate the beets whole at 95°F (35°C) until they lose 40–50 percent of their moisture (weigh before and after). The resulting food is a tough, gnarly little flavor bomb with a softer, delicious interior.

6. To serve, gently cut them into thin slices and arrange on a platter. Store in an airtight container in the fridge for up to 4 weeks.

●
FERMENTER'S NOTE

If you find the finished food too salty, you can drop the salt quantity to 1.75 percent, but no lower.

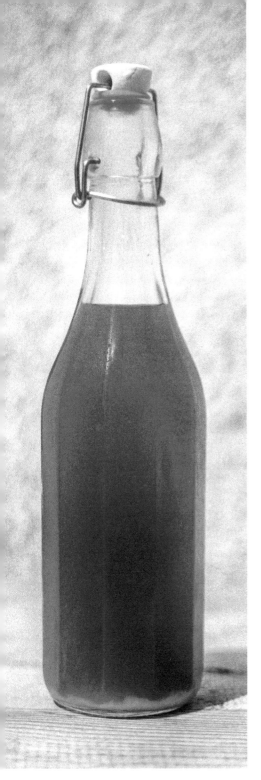

The range in color and flavor of homemade shoyu is staggering. This one turned out orange, but others come out golden, and some even deep black.

SPELT AND PEA SHOYU

Shoyu is the traditional Japanese soy sauce, distinct from other sauces thanks to the addition of wheat. In this version, I applied a home adaptation of shoyu to locally produced ingredients. Much like "peaso" is the pea-based version of miso, this shoyu swaps out soybeans for peas. I use a kind of stewing pea called carlin, which has a history in the North East of England, where my family is originally from. I also swapped out the traditional wheat for a locally grown spelt, but you can use any pea, bean, or corn from those listed in the applications chart (see p.175) and use wheat, spelt, rice, barley, or rye for a whole variety of flavors. When fully aged, this shoyu boasts an impressive savory umami flavor with notes of brioche. Unlike other kōji recipes in this book, shoyu is made by the direct application of spores on the prepared peas and spelt instead of combining with rice kōji.

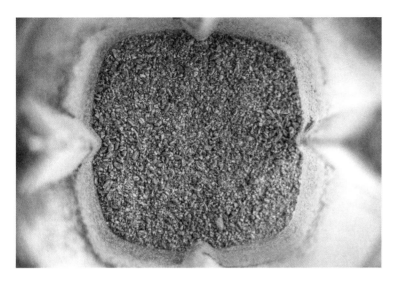
Step 5, coarsely pulsed spelt.

EQUIPMENT

canvas

powder shaker

probe thermometer

insulated box

hot-water bottle

3-liter jar

string or elastic band

cider press (optional)

INGREDIENTS

500g dried peas or beans

500g spelt

kōji spores (protease-specialized, such as *A. oryzae* or *A. sojae*)

1.6kg water

390g salt (15%)

1. Soak the peas overnight in 1 liter fresh cold water. The next day, drain them and leave for an hour in the open air to dry off.

2. Preheat the oven to 325°F (170°C) and spread the spelt out on a large, shallow baking sheet.

3. Put the sheet on the middle shelf of the oven and toast for an hour, stirring two or three times for even cooking.

4. Place the peas in a saucepan of fresh cold water. Bring to a gentle boil, cover with a lid, and continue to simmer until they're tender (as described in miso-making, p.191). This should take roughly 40–50 minutes, depending on the variety.

5. Coarsely mill the spelt, or use a food processor to pulse it two or three times. The aim here is to make a coarse meal, but not flour.

6. If all goes well, both peas and spelt will be ready at the same time. Drain the peas and spread them out on the canvas or a clean countertop. Add the spelt and mix them together, taking care not to burn yourself. Keep mixing until they've cooled enough to touch properly, roughly the temperature of a warm bath.

7. Use a powder shaker to inoculate with kōji spores, dusting a thin layer over the top, then mix the substrate and repeat the process. Do this three times to provide an even distribution.

8. Insert the probe and wrap the kōji mixture up in a damp dish towel, then wrap again in canvas. Place it in the insulated box (or the oven, turned off) and add the hot-water bottle to keep it warm. Secure the lid and leave for 12 hours. Monitor the temperature, and if it starts to drop below 86°F (30°C), refresh the hot-water bottle.

9. After 12 hours, unwrap the kōji mixture and break up the substrate. Rewrap it and continue to incubate for another 12 hours.

10. At 24 hours, place a rack inside a wooden, plastic, or nonreactive metal tray. Fill a heat-safe bowl with freshly boiled water and scald a clean dish towel in it for a minute. Carefully remove it and wring it out, then line the rack in the tray with the lightly dampened dish towel.

Below Step 7, inoculating freshly prepared peas and spelt with *A. oryzae* spores from a powder shaker.

Below right Step 11, shoyu substrate spread and furrowed, ready for the final growth phase. At this stage, the mixture smells strongly of jasmine.

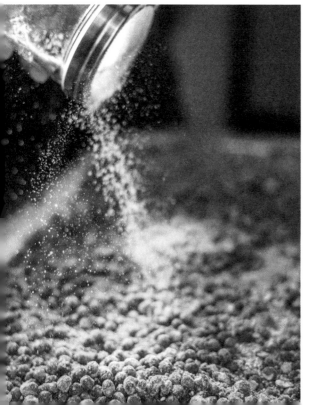

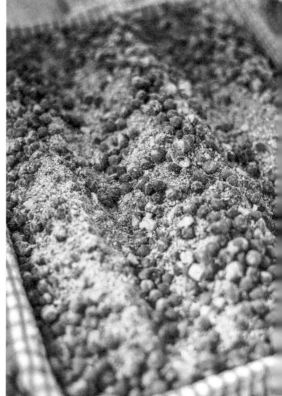

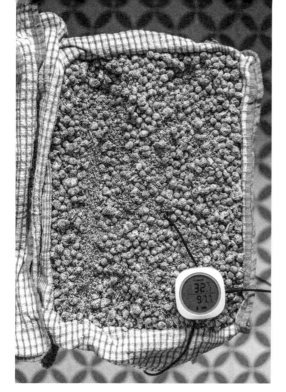
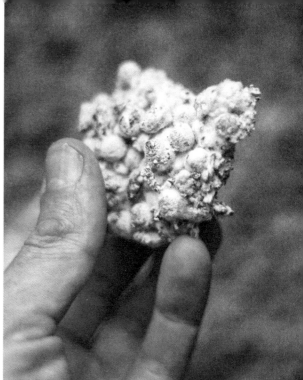

11. Spread the kōji out into the tray and form two furrows following the length of the tray, leaving a few centimeters clear at either end, as though plowing a field. Cover with a dry dish towel or untreated canvas and return to the insulated box for 24 hours. (A word of warning: depending on the depth of the kōji, this recipe can have a tendency to really take off and generate a lot of its own heat. Ideally, you want to keep it at 82–100°F/28–38°C, with a humidity above 80 percent. If you struggle to maintain this, spread the kōji more thinly between two trays.)

12. An hour before the kōji cycle is complete (47 hours), boil half the water, add it to the jar, and dissolve the salt. Add the remaining water to cool it down. Set aside until it reaches 86°F (30°C) or lower. After 48 hours, the kōji will have knitted the substrate together and formed a fine fuzz (especially over the peas). Feel free to crack one open and observe the mycelium growth inside. Break the kōji up and add it to the cooled salt water in the jar.

Above left Step 11, even uncovered and recently disturbed, the kōji remains above 88°F (31°C) and keeps its high humidity (important for umami flavors).

Above Step 12, a fully grown piece of shoyu kōji substrate, knitting together both pea and spelt.

13. Using a potato masher, rolling pin, or large spoon, stir and mash the kōji into the water for 30 seconds. Cover the surface with plastic wrap, secure a dish towel over the jar with string or an elastic band, and leave somewhere cool (64–72°F/18–22°C), out of direct sunlight.

14. For the first 2 weeks, open the shoyu up daily and give it a good stir. This is important, as it protects the mixture from going off and also aids the distribution of enzymes. After 2 weeks, this can be done once a week.

15. Age for 6–9 months, but taste it each week when you open it up to stir. As the flavor develops, a rich umami with subtle, sweet, fruity notes will appear.

16. If you have a cider press, line it and add the shoyu. Press it tightly to extract as much liquid as possible and leave the moromi behind (the paste that's left, see opposite). You could also try ice clarification (see p.189).

17. Shoyu should be stored in a bottle in the fridge for up to 1 year. Shoyu can be pasteurized in a water bath at 185°F (85°C) for 8 minutes, but only if you have filtered all the sediment out. Pasteurizing will alter the aroma and flavor of shoyu but will make it stable at room temperature.

FERMENTER'S NOTE

If it tastes mushroomy, chances are your kōji ran to spore. While this isn't a bad taste, it can muddy a pure shoyu. To avoid this, catch the kōji a little earlier next time when adding it to the brine.

Freshly prepared shoyu in salt water (left) and 9 months later (right).

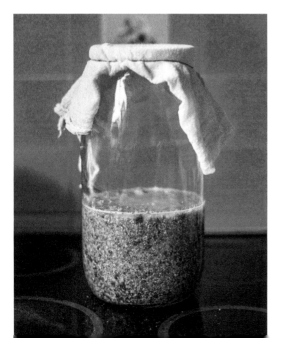

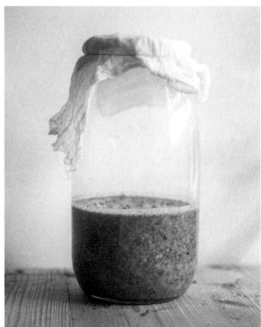

MOROMI

If you don't like the idea of waste, you can use moromi as a seasoning in a similar capacity to miso. Either store it in an airtight container in the fridge for up to 1 month or dehydrate it at 113°F (45°C) for 12–14 hours and grind it into a flour to use as a deeply umami powder, perfect for adding in stews, dumpling fillings, sauces, or mixing into flour to dust fried foods. Once you've pressed the shoyu from moromi, collect it in a bottle and store in the fridge. It will last up to 9 months, but it should always be kept in the fridge (as should any artisan soy sauce or shoyu, once opened) to slow the deterioration that takes place once the aging passes its peak.

COOKING WITH FERMENTS

CURED YOLKS

Mix 4 parts shoyu to 1 part mirin, then gently add egg yolks. Cover and cure in the fridge for 10 hours. Serve on rice or in salads.

BROTHS, SOUPS, AND SAUCES

Give body, depth, and umami to broths, soups, and stock. Use as the base to both teriyaki and gyoza dipping sauce.

GLAZE

Brush shoyu over rice and fish.

SALT REPLACEMENT

Use in almost any recipe in place of salt to complement sweet and savory.

SHOYU VARIATIONS

Shoyu doesn't have to be made with beans or peas—it can also be made with corn.

CORN SHOYU

For corn shoyu (where corn replaces beans or peas), boil the corn with cal (cal mexicana, slaked lime, or calcium hydroxide). This chemical is used by the food industry, throughout many traditional Asian cuisines, but also specifically by the Aztecs in preparation of maize. The alkaline cal makes corn more digestible and tasty, perfect for fermentation. To do so, add 5g chef-grade calcium hydroxide per 500g of corn (1 percent). Cover with cold water 2in (5cm) above the level of the corn, cover with a lid, and bring to a boil. Reduce to a simmer and cook for an hour. Once cooked, leave covered to soak for 8–12 hours, then wash the corn under fresh cold water. This process will remove the hull, which will have come loose during cooking. Once it's removed, the corn is now ready to grind and inoculate with kōji spores.

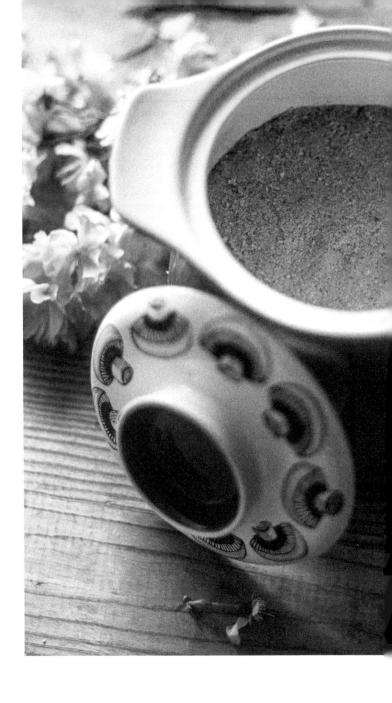

NUKAZUKE

A nukadoko is a changing, living
thing that can smell umami, sour,
and yeasty as it matures.

You can think of nukazuke as a unique style of pickling that
uses solid-state fermentation. A combination of three main
types of microbes, it truly epitomizes lessons from each of
the chapters in this book. Unlike pickling using just vinegar
or lacto fermentation, a nukadoko (the rice bran fermenting
"bed" of the nukazuke) harnesses the enzymes and flavors
of yeasts, kōji, lactic acid bacteria, and—a new player to
this book—butyric acid bacteria. This rare bacteria is
uncommon in foods, but the acid it produces is very good
for gut health. The most famous food you'll recognize its
characteristic flavor and smell from is none other than
Parmesan cheese. And a freshly pickled vegetable from a
nukazuke has distinct Parmesan notes.

Once made, a nukazuke requires daily mixing to
maintain a constant and healthy biome, along with regular
feeds of fresh produce. This process can be slowed by
storing it in the fridge, but for the best results, keep it at
room temperature. We mix the nukadoko because of the
unique characteristics of each different microbe within it
and the different areas they occupy. Yeasts, which love
oxygen, live on the surface, while LAB thrive in the middle.
At the deepest, darkest area at the bottom, we find the
butyric acid bacteria, thriving in the absence of oxygen.
A nukazuke becomes more stable in time. Mine was made
with a small amount of a nukadoko first started by Haruko's
grandfather over 60 years ago. So, in the tradition of
fermentation starters, I named it after him, 大有 (Taiyu).
Setting up a nukadoko doesn't require inoculation from
a mature batch, but this will help stabilize the ferment
more quickly.

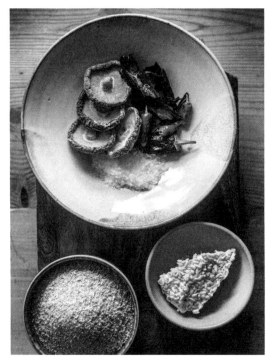

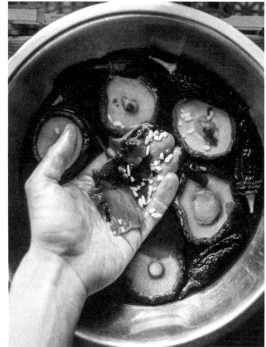

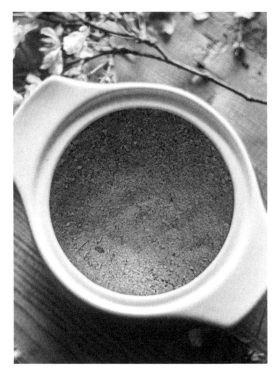

Above left All the ingredients
of a nukadoko.

Above right Soaking the
ingredients in water to infuse
flavor and enzymes.

Left A freshly prepared
nukadoko in a ceramic crock.

fermentation crock

INGREDIENTS

500g water

3 dried chili peppers

3 dried shiitake mushrooms

1 tbsp seaweed (kombu or dulse)

5 tbsp rice kōji (see p.166)

500g rice bran, wheat bran, or oat bran

50g salt (5%)

vegetables, such as cabbage and carrot

1. Pour the water over the chilies, mushrooms, seaweed, and rice kōji (ideally, the water should be around 41°F/5°C) and leave to infuse for 2 hours.

2. Add the liquid, with all the ingredients except for the mushrooms, into the rice bran to make a thick oatmeal, then add the salt and mix thoroughly. (You can cook and eat the mushrooms now they have done their job infusing the water.)

3. Transfer the nukadoko into a clean fermentation crock. To set off fermentation, add some fresh, clean vegetables. A few cabbage leaves and a carrot will do. Bury them below the surface of the rice bran.

USING THE NUKADOKO

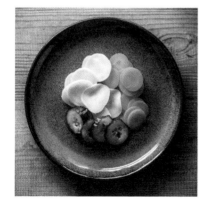

Radish, carrot, and cucumber pickled for 24 hours in a nukadoko.

Before pickling ingredients, sprinkle over salt to draw out excess moisture and leave for 30 minutes. Then wash and pat dry before burying in the rice bran. Pickling like this can be as quick as 30 minutes or as long as a week. I advise you to dig up your vegetables from the rice bran at different times and cut a thin slice off. Taste to see how the flavor has developed and decide if you wish to age further.

As you use the nukadoko regularly, moisture from the vegetables will eventually start to flood the rice bran. When this happens, simply add equal parts rice bran and water, mixed with salt (5 percent of the weight of both the bran and water combined) to counter the moisture. Alternative grain brans can also be used, so have fun and find something that's grown in your area.

If you're going away for a while or wish to slow down the nukadoko for less frequent use, store it in the fridge, where it will need mixing and feeding once a week or so. If left for too long without stirring, it can develop a powdery kahm yeast on the surface. This might look bad, but it can be scooped off and discarded with no long-lasting damage to the nukadoko, which, when looked after, can last forever.

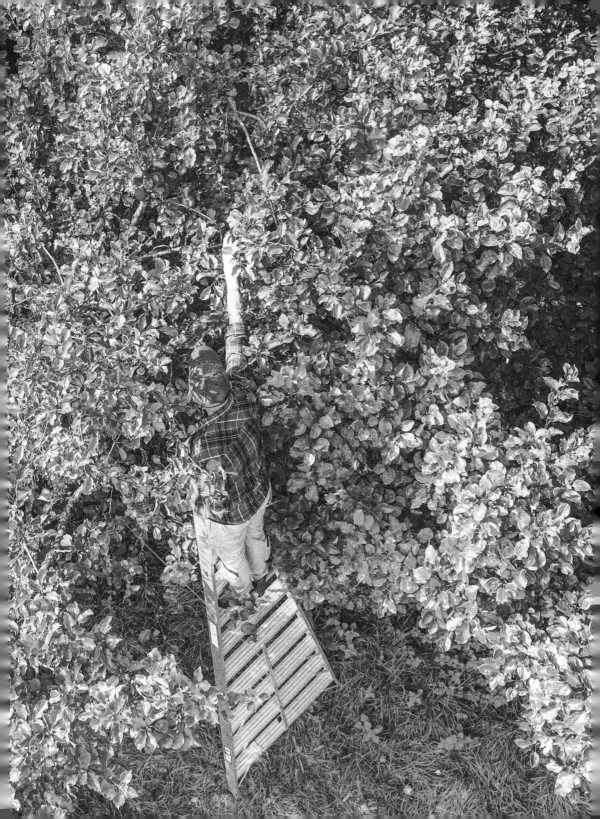

TROUBLE-SHOOTING

Sometimes, despite doing everything right, fermentation doesn't always go how we'd like. Some problems can be countered; others cannot (and for the sake of safety, they must be discarded and started again). In this section, I'll cover what to look out for and how to stay on the right side of that line.

It is perfectly normal for the colors of ingredients to change and fade, even bleed out into the water and juices surrounding them during fermentation. Liquids will turn cloudy; sediment will gather at the bottom of the vessel; and if you're lucky, you might even make your own alien-looking vinegar mother. The whole process can feel a bit unnerving if you're new to it—it can sometimes feel unnerving for a seasoned professional! As I mentioned before, remember to trust your nose and sense of smell. It is normal for ferments to have powerful aromas, but if something smells bad, throw it out.

INACTIVITY

When a ferment doesn't spring into life, it's usually a sign that the temperature is a little too cold. This will slow the microorganisms or even put them into a dormant state. I find the ideal temperature is 68–77°F (20–25°C). While lactic acid bacteria (LAB) will thrive at temperatures up to 104°F (40°C) and most yeasts up to 95°F (35°C), I find the hotter range induces overly active ferments, which produce thinner, shallow flavors. For the same reason cider is made in fall, riding that fine line between a slow, cold temperature and a too-cold (dormant) temperature can yield complex, delicious results. However, if your ferment does nothing, try

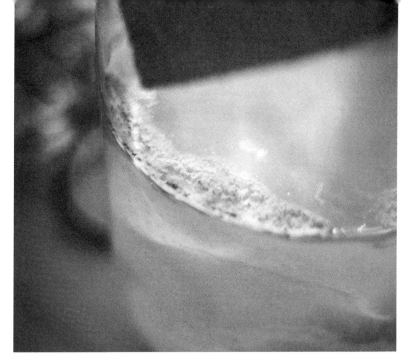

Mold growth on the surface of a dried SCOBY in kombucha.

moving it somewhere warmer. If it still doesn't creep into life, open the lid and give it a stir to disturb the liquid and ingredients. This will redistribute the ingredients and introduce oxygen into the liquid, giving the microbes a boost. You can also turn to those fermentation heroes, garlic and ginger (see p.28).

For mold, pay attention to the temperature ranges in the recipe and the use-by date on the tane kōji packet. I find kōji spores perform well for 6 months after opening, as long as you keep them stored in a fridge, sealed in an airtight bag. After this, performance becomes sporadic.

FALSE STARTS

Sometimes a ferment will launch into action, then inexplicably stop after just a few days. There are many reasons for this, but the most effective fix is to remove the lid and give it a really good stir—stir it so that you create a vortex swirling in the container. The aim here is to introduce oxygen into the fermenting liquid and kick-start the microbes into action again. Then put the lid back on and wait a day or two.

KAHM YEAST

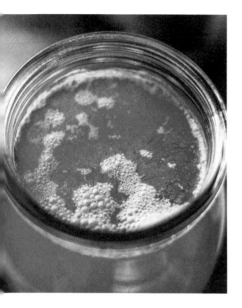

Kahm yeast starting to form on the surface of a sugary ferment.

The harmless bane of fermenters everywhere, kahm is a foul-tasting, off-white or greenish powdery yeast that can grow on the surface of both liquid and solid ferments. One of the best counters is to lay food-safe plastic, plastic wrap, or parchment paper over the surface of the ferment long before kahm ever appears. This blocks direct contact with oxygen and stops kahm from growing, although it can still appear at the edges.

If kahm has already appeared, use a clean spoon to carefully scoop it away. The sooner you catch this, the less affected the flavor of your ferment will be. Discard the kahm and wipe down the insides of the jar or crock with a paper towel doused with white vinegar. Lay a fresh piece of parchment or plastic wrap over the surface and return the jar to its fermenting location. Keep an eye on it over the next few days in case the yeast returns around the edges of the parchment and repeat the process if required.

Sometimes kōji-based recipes will produce a white or off-white layer on top. This can be kahm yeast or kōji. (You can usually smell the difference.) If you're suspicious it's kahm, remove it as described above. If it's kōji, it won't do any damage and can be left alone.

To reiterate, kahm is completely harmless. Nothing bad will happen if you accidentally eat some, and it won't turn your ferment toxic. It just tastes awful.

GOLDILOCKS FIZZ

One of the most common questions I get asked about is people either struggling to make their drinks carbonated or scared of bottles and jars exploding from too much carbonation. As mentioned before in this book, one way to practice gauging this is to use a plastic bottle so you can feel how much pressure is building up, then you can transfer the same timings to glass bottles. You can also set off multiple bottles of one large ferment and sacrifice one after a day or two to see how the whole batch is progressing.

As a general guide, if you bottle an active ferment such as kombucha, ginger beer, or ale in a 1-liter bottle with

1–2 teaspoons of additional sugar, hold it at 77°F (25°C) for 24–36 hours, then chill in a fridge for 12–24 hours. You should have a pleasantly sparkling beverage—not too fizzy, and not too flat.

When it comes to jars, we almost never want carbonation. Sure, it looks fun, but in the case of miso and amino pastes, carbonation has a detrimental effect on flavors. For other ferments, we don't want oxygen, but we equally aren't after carbonation either. You can keep on top of things by burping the jars daily, opening the lid to release the pressure, then sealing it again. If you're going away or don't trust yourself to remember, use an elastic band as a makeshift airlock (see p.67) or self-burping jar. Or you can get a lid with an built-in valve or airlock.

MISO PROBLEMS

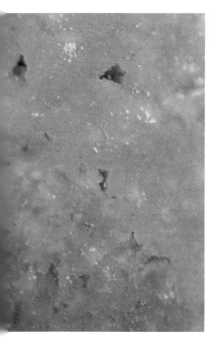

Tyrosine crystals forming in miso.

Sometimes miso will develop cracks running through it that can lead to mold growth. This is why the correct moisture content and packing techniques are so important. If mold grows into your miso, despite it sometimes looking like *Aspergillus* (white and fluffy), chances are it isn't. (*Aspergillus* cannot tolerate such a salty environment.) If this happens, I advise you to start over, as there's no telling how dangerous an unknown mold could be.

If your miso smells alcoholic, then there is too much moisture in the mixture, allowing yeasts to ferment the sugars produced by kōji from substrate starches.

If using a jar for miso, you may notice tiny white specks appearing against the glass. These are most likely a type of amino acid crystal (tyrosine), which form when proteins break down. Most commonly found in hard cheeses, these are a natural part of aging.

FURTHER READING

- *The Art of Fermentation*, Sandor Katz
- *Baking School,* Justin Gellatly, Louise Gellatly, Matthew Jones
- *The Flavour Thesaurus*, Niki Segnit
- *The Forager's Calendar*, John Wright
- *Koji Alchemy*, Jeremy Umansky, Rich Shih
- *The Larousse Book of Bread*, Éric Kayser
- *The Noma Guide to Fermentation*, René Redzepi and David Zilber
- *Preserving the Japanese Way*, Nancy Singleton Hachisu
- *Salt, Fat, Acid, Heat*, Samin Nosrat
- *The Self-Sufficiency Garden*, Huw Richards and Sam Cooper (should you wish to grow your own ingredients to ferment).
- *Tartine Bread* by Chad Robertson
- *Tasting History,* Max Miller
- *Wildcrafted Fermentation*, Pascal Baudar

RESOURCES

- Excalibur for dehydrator
- Inkbird Bluetooth Temperature and Humidity Sensor (there are also Wi-Fi models available that are useful)
- Inkbird or Brewing Mate heating pads for hands-off temperature control
- Kilner for jars and glassware
- Kōji spores: The Koji Fermenteria (UK); Hakko.online (USA); Koji & Co (AUS); or follow me @chef.sam. black for more supplier information
- Sous Vide Tools for vacuum machines

INDEX

ACKNOWLEDGMENTS

In no particular order... My family and Wai Yan for your support and patience; Cara, Lucy, and Jordan, as well as the rest of the wonderful team at DK; Huw Richards for giving me the time, encouragement, and ingredients to make this book possible; Haruko Uchishiba of The Koji Fermenteria for teaching me the traditions of kōji and continuing to be a source of inspiration and guidance; Jihyun Kim of Kimchi & Radish for your insight, enthusiasm, and experience in kimchi making; Kilner for kindly supplying the equipment to ferment a book's worth of food; Sous Vide Tools for kindly offering a chamber sealer and compostable pouches for this project; James Weiss for the use of his wonderful microscopic images of yeast and bacteria; and to every single person who makes up the weird and wonderful community of foodies and fermenters online – you share so much and I am forever grateful.

ABOUT THE AUTHOR

Sam Cooper is a chef, fermenter, photographer, illustrator, and gardener. He began working in kitchens before meeting gardener Huw Richards and becoming co-director for Regenerative Media. He has a following of 570,000+ as @chef.sam.black on Instagram, where he shares videos using homegrown, seasonal, and foraged produce to unlock incredible flavors by fermentation. Sam and Huw's book *The Self-sufficiency Garden* was a number-one *Sunday Times* bestseller in 2024, and his debut book *The Nature of Food* published in 2022.

Publisher acknowledgments

DK would like to thank Kathryn Glendenning for proofreading and Ruth Ellis for indexing.

Picture credits

The publisher would like to thank the following for their kind permission to reproduce their photographs:

James Weiss: 2, 4

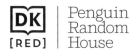

Editorial Director Cara Armstrong
Project Editor Lucy Philpott
US Senior Editor Kayla Dugger
US Executive Editor Lori Cates Hand
Project Art Editor Jordan Lambley
DTP and Design Co-ordinator Heather Blagden
Production Editor David Almond
Senior Production Controller Stephanie McConnell
Jacket Designer Jordan Lambley
Jacket and Sales Material Co-ordinator Emily Cannings
Art Director Maxine Pedliham

Editor Kate Reeves-Brown
Designer Nikki Ellis

First American Edition, 2024
Published in the United States by DK Publishing,
a division of Penguin Random House LLC
1745 Broadway, 20th Floor, New York, NY 10019

A catalog record for this book
is available from the Library of Congress.
ISBN 978-0-5938-4789-3

DK books are available at special discounts when purchased in bulk for sales promotions, premiums, fund-raising, or educational use. For details, contact: DK Publishing Special Markets, 1745 Broadway, 20th Floor, New York, NY 10019
SpecialSales@dk.com

Printed and bound in Slovakia

www.dk.com

MIX
Paper | Supporting responsible forestry
FSC
www.fsc.org
FSC™ C018179

This book was made with Forest Stewardship Council™ certified paper—one small step in DK's commitment to a sustainable future. Learn more at www.dk.com/uk/information/sustainability